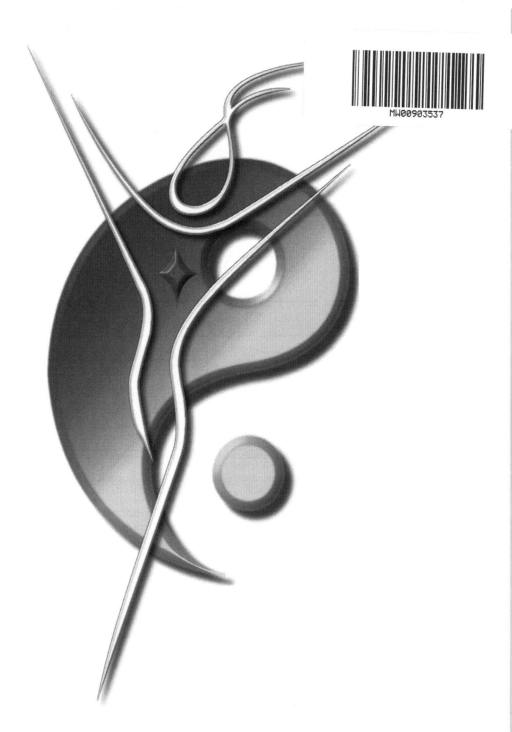

BALANCED

The "Balanced Body Type"
is symbolized by the Yin/Yang symbol.
Dependent upon everything working together
synergistically, Balanced body types need balance
between work and play, as well as all other aspects
of life. Essentially playful and adventurous,
they embody the synergy that
brings about balance.

The Ideal Diet — *Does It Exist?*

An *ideal* diet is the one that nutritionally supports *your* specific dietary requirements. It's a way of eating that optimizes your health and vitality as well as normalizing your weight. Most diets are based on the myth that "One Diet Fits All." Many people think that if they can't stay on a diet, it's because they lack willpower. The reality is your body will have food cravings when it doesn't get the nutrients it needs.

The problem with most diets is that they are too general and do not address the specific needs of the individual such as "What time of day do I eat fruit or protein and which vegetables do I eat?" One diet does *not* fit all. Each person has a dominant gland, organ, or system that is stronger than the others which determines weight gain patterns, physical characteristics, and food cravings. This "dominant" gland is the basis of *The 25 Body Type System*™.

Look to *The 25 Body Type System*™ for the diet that truly supports your specific nutritional needs. Following your ideal diet will optimize your health and vitality as well as normalize your weight. Inability to maintain your ideal weight is the first sign of the body being out of balance. *Different Bodies, Different Diets*™ gives you the dietary guidance to optimize your health.

BALANCED PROFILE & DIET

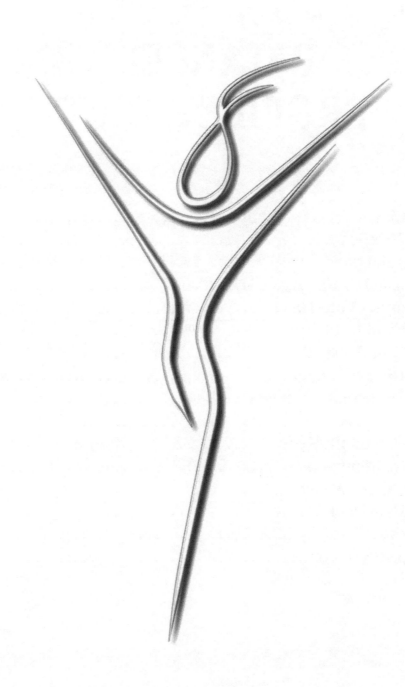

Explanation of Terms and Format

Location & Function

Provides the location and function of the gland, organ or system associated with each body type. The location is where, when healthy, the majority of the body's energy resides and, when depleted, where the body is most vulnerable.

Potential Health Problems

Identifies the problems your body type is prone to develop when your dominant gland becomes exhausted; includes early warning signs.

Recommended Exercise

Anaerobic exercise is essential for some body types, as it activates the immune system. Surprisingly, this isn't true for all body types. Some types are better with aerobic exercise such as yoga or Tai Chi since this type of exercise serves to rebuild the energy in the body. While exercise has many physical benefits, for most people, its greatest significance is in bringing about emotional well-being. Emotional benefits include releasing stress, clearing or calming the mind, and getting energy moving.

Exercise doesn't have to *"look"* like exercise. Ordinary daily activities can provide the needed movement required by some types. Included in this exercise section are the types of exercises that provide the greatest benefits.

One of the easiest ways to incorporate exercise is to use the Fitness Ball as a chair. Sitting on the ball forces you to use your pelvic and lower abdominal muscles. This improves posture and stimulates cerebral-spinal fluid movement, resulting in increased alertness and mental clarity.

Distinguishing Features

These features alone can often be sufficient to differentiate one body type from another. However, not every member of a type necessarily has them, or to the degree where they are strongly evident.

Additional Physical Characteristics

Supplementary characteristics are useful for comparing and contrasting different body types. Since physical characteristics reflect ethnic and familial heritage as well as dominant and sub-dominant gland characteristics, they can vary considerably. I've described the characteristics that are most commonly seen within each type and noted the ones that tend to run the entire range. For example, height in **Liver** types can vary from very petite to very tall, even though the majority is of average height. So, *don't rule out a type simply because one or two characteristics don't apply to you.*

Weight Gain Areas

Women: The initial weight gain pattern provides the most important—and often the simplest and most obvious criterion—for determining a woman's body type. Secondary gain refers to any weight gain over 15 pounds.

Men: Describes weight gain as to location and musculature appearance, including areas of primary and secondary weight gain.

Scheduling Meals

A quick guide for choosing which foods to eat for breakfast, lunch, and dinner, and your ideal meal times.

Choose from the ***Healthy*** list when you feel strong and healthy, with plenty of energy available to digest your food.

Choose from the ***Sensitive*** list when your body is under stress (either physical, mental or emotional). During these times, energy has been directed elsewhere and is less available for digestion.

Dietary Emphasis

Gives recommendations for weight loss or gain. Lists fat and protein requirements and their best sources. Fats supply essential fatty acids, but not all fats qualify to be included in the minimum fat requirement. Vegetarian diets support some body types, but not all.

Foods High in Amino Acids

Lists the highest sources that are most easily assimilated for your body type. The amino acids threonine, isoleucine and cystine are depleted when a person goes through a lot of changes or personal growth.

Key Supports for System

Suggests foods and/or activities to optimally strengthen or support your particular body type.

Complementary Glandular Support

Identifies the two glands needing to be rebuilt or supported that will give your dominant gland a rest; suggests how this is best accomplished.

Foods Craved

(When Energy is Low) Lists the foods that, by stimulating the body's dominant gland, provide the greatest immediate, but temporary, energy lift.

Foods to Avoid

Identifies foods that are particularly difficult for your body to assimilate, or ones that cause excessive stress.

Recommended Cuisine

The cuisine most supportive to your system—particularly useful when you're dining out and need to select the most appropriate restaurant. Also included are the foods best suited to your type on a daily basis.

Psychological Profile

The Essence embodies the basic nature of each body type. The profile is often the deciding factor in body type identification. Relying on food preferences is often unreliable, since the desire for supporting foods can shift when the dominant gland becomes depleted. Psychological characteristics are often observed from birth and can be useful in identifying a child's body type.

Becoming familiar with the personality parameters of the various body types can help you gain insight into your own personal strengths and challenges, as well as expand your self-awareness. Additionally, aside from better understanding your own basic nature, increasing your knowledge about the psychological dimensions of the other body types can enhance your understanding and acceptance of others different from you.

**Phychological
Profile (cont.)**

Greater awareness and understanding of yourself provides compassion and understanding of yourself and others. Being aware of the foods you eat and the effect they have on your body is often the first step in self-awareness.

Emotional Issues

While we all have all the emotional patterns, there are some issues that are more of a problem for some types than others. The emotional issues that create the greatest stress are the basic learning challenges for each body type and are listed here along with the other side of the emotion and the affirmation or way of shifting a negative emotional experience to a positive one.

Clearing an emotional pattern is achieved most quickly by connecting and releasing all aspects: the emotional, mental, physical and spiritual.

Feeling both sides of the emotion provides a focus and gives the blocked emotion a positive direction in which to move. Knowing both sides of the emotion allows for a mental understanding and brings the experience into a conscious awareness.

The spiritual aspect is achieved by the transition statement which provides a means of moving from the negative to the positive side of the emotion.

Essential oils access the limbic system of the brain which is the seat of emotion. When essential oils are applied to the alarm points, the cellular memory stored in the body is released.

To clear an emotion, smell the essential oil, feel both sides of the emotion, say the transition statement and apply the appropriate essential oil to the associated alarm point and the emotional release points on the frontal eminences of the forehead. Repeat as needed—whenever the emotion arises or you think about it, as well as at night before going to sleep.

More information is available in ***Releasing Emotional Patterns with Essential Oils,*** also by Carolyn L. Mein, D.C. *(see Body Type Products at the end of this book for a list of the Oils book and other Body Typing publications).*

Physical Profile

Location	All over, since no one gland is in charge.
Function	With Balanced types, all glands, organs, and systems must work together harmoniously for optimal functioning.
Potential Health Problems	Headaches, either tension or migraine (frequently relieved by caffeine); neck and shoulder tension; digestive distress, such as indigestion, constipation, intestinal inflammation; food allergies (may be hidden); hypoglycemia; kidney or bladder infections; and menstrual distress. May experience weakness or hyperactivity due to low blood sugar if meals are skipped.
Recommended Exercise	The initial benefit of exercise for the Balanced body type is emotional. It gets energy moving, lifts spirits, adds variety to daily activities, and activates the physical body by getting the lymphatics moving. Sunlight is beneficial, and being around water is often important. Variety is essential. Exercise may include Pilates, dancing, walking, hiking, bicycling, swimming, rebounding, weight lifting, baseball, or tennis.

Women's Characteristics

Distinguishing Features	Buttocks somewhat flat, due to blending into upper and outer thighs, creating a rather droopy appearance. Bright, sparkling eyes – especially when smiling. Essentially playful and adventurous, they embody the synergy that brings about balance.
Additional Physical Characteristics	Rounded-to-prominent buttocks that appear flat. Low back curvature average-to-swayed. Breasts small-to-average. Shoulders relatively even with, to broader than, hips. Defined waist. Long-waisted with short-to-average legs, or short-waisted with long legs. Height generally average, but can range from petite to tall. Bone structure small-to-medium. Average, elongated musculature. Hands average-to-broad, square palm with square or short fingers, characterized by wide reach. Good joint flexibility. May have had long arms as child, sometimes also as adult. Average oval or rectangular face with high forehead, or heart-shaped, pixie-like face with V-shaped chin.
Women's Weight Gain Areas	Lower body with initial gain in entire upper 2/3rds of thighs extending into lower buttocks, upper inner thighs, lower abdomen, minimally in waist, upper and/or lower hips. Secondary gain in entire thighs, eventually extending into entire abdomen, middle back, upper arms, and upper hips.

Physical Profile

Men's Characteristics

Distinguishing Features

Often long-waisted with long torso and short legs, or short torso with long legs. May have wide hips. Balance is essential. Basic nature is gentle, playful and adventurous. Music or creativity is an intrinsic part of life. Precise analytical mind coupled with a gentle demeanor.

Additional Physical Characteristics

Buttocks relatively flat to prominent. Low back curvature straight-to-average. Shoulders relatively even with, to moderatel broader than, hips. Average, proportionate torso with average musculature. Moderate ability to attain muscle definition in torso. Natural lower abdominal protrusion or lower-to-entire paunch. Average-to-muscular thighs and calves. Height ranges from average to very tall. Bone structure medium. Average hands, characterized by wide reach and good flexibility. Average neck. Average oval or rectangular face with high forehead, or heart-shaped face with V-shaped chin. Hair generally full, of average thickness. Hair loss pattern is frontal with hairline receding straight back causing a rising forehead, or minimal at upper sides. Physical characteristics show strong secondary gland influence, such as solid musculature of Adrenal type, or low forehead and heavy eyebrows of Medulla.

Men's Weight Gain Areas

Initial gain in lower-to-entire abdomen as solid musculature and around waist as solid thickening. May have soft layer of fat covering abdomen. Secondary gain as lower-to-entire abdominal paunch, solid thickening or soft rolls at waist, minimal thickening in torso, hips, buttocks, thighs, and under chin.

**Scheduling
"Healthy" Meals**

*Schedule **Healthy** meals when you feel strong and healthy, with plenty of energy available to digest your food.*

Breakfast: Light-to-moderate, with grain and/or fruit, vegetables, dairy, nuts, and/or seeds. Emphasize carbohydrates, with moderate fats.

Lunch: Moderate, with protein, grain, vegetables, and/or dairy. Emphasize protein.

Dinner: Moderate, with grain, vegetables, legumes, protein, and/or dairy. Emphasize grain and vegetables.

Dietary Emphasis

• *Balance* raw and cooked vegetables.

• *For weight loss,* avoid caffeine, stimulants (including Ma Haung and alcohol), and sugar; derive no more than 25-30% of caloric intake from fats (if fats fall below 20%, weight will stabilize); limit portion size; eat light dinner, consuming majority of calories at breakfast and lunch; eat fruit only for breakfast; avoid snacking after dinner; delete starches (especially breads and grains with wheat) at dinner; reduce dairy; and rotate foods. Emphasize protein and vegetables with 15% of caloric intake from dense protein. To keep weight off, especially important to lose it slowly.

• *For weight gain,* increase protein when underweight; if at ideal weight or above, sugar, including dried fruit and honey, and dairy, especially ice cream and milk, will add extra pounds.

• *Vegetarian diets inadequate,* since Balanced types require 10-30% of calories from dense protein.

• Fats, 20-30% of caloric intake, should be derived from butter and dense protein (chicken, turkey, eggs, fish, beef).

**Foods High
in Amino Acids**

• When going through a lot of changes or personal growth, the amino acids threonine, isoleucine, and cystine are depleted. They are highest and most easily assimilated in tuna, sunflower seeds and ricotta cheese.

**Key Support for
System**

Rotation essential – ideally, allow four days before repeating food. Balance choices from all food groups.

Dietary Guidelines

Complementary Glandular Support

Thyroid, through consuming two oz. of dense protein (chicken, turkey, eggs, or fish) with grain, such as rice or pasta, five times weekly; and pancreas, through rotating foods.

Foods Craved

(When Energy is Low) Sweets (pastries, cookies, chocolate – especially Reese's™ peanut butter cups); fruit (strawberries as child); carbohydrates (popcorn, white and wheat breads, hoagie sandwich, pizza); fats; or salty foods like chips, processed meats; drinks with caffeine.

Foods to Avoid

Any food that is a problem for you. Some of the more common ones are: raw onions, because they can cause indigestion; chocolate, because it can raise blood pressure; cookies, because they can raise body heat excessively, even to point of facial flushing; sugar, because it can cause fatigue or sleep disturbances; wheat or yeast, because they can cause sleepiness or loss of mental focus. Leg pain may result from certain food combinations, such as carrot/celery/beet juice. In general, search out food sensitivities (which can come from any food group) and eliminate.

Recommended Cuisine

Chinese, Thai, Sushi, Japanese, Moroccan, Mexican, French, Indian. Foods moderately seasoned, protein and grain combinations.

Psychological Profile

Essence

Just as the Balanced body type is not controlled by any single gland, organ or system, but is dependent upon everything working together synergistically, Balanced body types need balance in their world. This means balance between work and play, physical and spiritual expression, mental and emotional states, and relationships, both personal and business. In other words, balance in both their inner and outer worlds, between people and life in general. Essentially playful and adventurous, they embody the synergy that brings about balance.

Characteristic Traits

Sensitive by nature, Balanced types have a fragile equilibrium and will go to great lengths to maintain their delicate balance. On the outside, they are often light, playful, personable and entertaining, while being reserved on the inside, reluctant to share their true feelings. Generally quite social, people are readily attracted to them but rarely allowed to get very close emotionally until they've proven that they can be trusted.

Balanced body types have a strong sense of adventure and like to travel or move frequently, giving them the opportunity to meet new people and try new things. They love performing or being the center of attention, and since they are typically in their glory when interacting with people, will often be the life of the party. They mix well with others and can be quite good at making favorable impressions. They are basically easygoing, forgiving, optimistic, and open-minded individuals, with a positive attitude toward life.

Adventure is what creates an aliveness and a love of life that is often expressed as new ideas, concepts and designs. Imaginative and creative, with a strong attraction to the Arts, Balanced types have a need for order and structure that allows them to be extremely precise in their music, dance or creative expression. Sensitive and artistic, they are also practical, logical, and technically adept. Their acute sense of sight, hearing and touch is balanced with a natural sense of rhythm and timing which they often use to discover their inner sense of stability and balance.

Motivation

Because of their extreme sensitivity to imbalances, Balanced types have a heightened need for security and stability, causing them to go to great lengths to control their environment. They need to work in situations that ensure maximum predictability and harmony. They often find it difficult to delegate tasks or supervise others and feel that it's faster and more effective to do a job personally. Consequently, they prefer to work alone, taking full responsi-bility for the outcome and offering their personal guarantee that the job will be done right. By working alone they also avoid the unpleasant task of criticizing or correcting co-workers.

Psychological Profile

Despite the care they take in projecting a positive image, Balanced types are known to undermine their own efforts. For example, by placing such a high value on honesty, truthfulness can override diplomacy and result in tactless comments. There is a tendency to speak without censoring words. They have difficulty keeping secrets and don't like others to be secretive, often becoming very impatient when others withhold information.

Being intuitively aware of the dangers relationships pose, and taking commitments seriously, they are cautious about making them. Consequently, as a protective mechanism, they may have a fear of intimacy, which compels them to distance themselves from others and limit close friends to a select few. They need to develop relationships slowly and to know others well, before they are willing to reveal their innermost thoughts and feelings.

"At Worst"

Balanced types can become extremely impatient both with themselves and others when things go wrong and their need for order and balance isn't satisfied. Unless they've developed considerable self-control, they may display anger or even rage, and then regret it later. They can overreact with rigidity and intolerance or retreat from problems through compulsive/addictive behavior in the form of an activity, a relationship, or substance abuse.

If they haven't developed an inner sense of stability, Balanced types will typically look to others to provide it. Since relationships can never fulfill what can only come from within, expecting to gain stability from outer relationships makes them prone to disillusionment, or settling for relationships that are detrimental to their personal growth and inner peace.

Motivated by the need for acceptance by others, Balanced types will often suppress or even deny their feelings, causing them to appear distant, detached, or preoccupied. Their fear of rejection can cause them to keep their feelings hidden to avoid upsetting themselves or others. These suppressed emotions generally surface as physical complaints, like headaches or digestive problems. Balanced types use play and adventurous activities to release stored-up emotional energy. When out of balance, they can get so caught up in their play and fantasies that they lose sight of reality.

Psychological Profile

"At Best"

Balanced types are persistent, goal-oriented self-starters who like to be in control of their work, gladly accepting responsibility for the completion of a task. They are good at seeing to the heart of a matter, focusing more on the big picture or the main objective than on technicalities, so as not to be distracted by surface appearances. While they are not primarily detail-oriented, they'll make sure the details are correct before finally releasing a project. Conscientious and competent, they can be depended upon to fulfill their promises and are often found working late into the night to finish a project.

Engaging in adventurous activities and daring pursuits that capture the imagination and challenge their problem solving abilities allows Balanced types to get rid of pent-up stress and revitalize themselves through play. They find the balance between work and play by finding their passion and making work and play synonymous. Balancing work with play helps them find the harmony they need for a sense of well-being. This in turn helps them maintain an optimistic, open-minded, positive attitude toward life enabling them to bounce back from adversity.

Having developed their intuitive nature, they are guided by their deep sense of stability and balance, causing them to create positive experiences in relationships and in life overall. By solidly connecting with their spiritual center and developing their own stability, they are able to establish a nurturing relationship with themselves, and break free from their fears and self-imposed restrictions. By discovering their deeper truths and movements, they are able to live more from the potential that each day and each moment offers.

Balanced types are self-contained and at peace within themselves. Having developed an inner sense of harmony and balance, they have an easygoing, forgiving, and humorous nature that brings a lightness and balance into the lives of those they touch.

Psychological Profile

Emotional Issues

Emotional issues that are basic lessons for the Balanced body type are the *fear of losing control, fear of rejection,* and *feeling of "F—You".*

The higher octave of **control** is *balance.* The transitional statement is *"I am content and blessed."* The fear of control is stored in the stomach. The alarm point is on both sides near the sternum, between the breast. The essential oil, **Peace & Calming**, is used to release the need to control and is applied to the stomach alarm points and the emotional points on the frontal eminences.

The other side of **rejection** (fear of being rejected) is *acceptance.* The transitional statement is *"I accept all that I am."* Fear of being rejected is stored in the lungs. The alarm points are on the front of the body, the upper chest just above the armpit, in two inches, toward the center of the body and one inch below the clavicle. The essential oil, **Purification**, is applied to the lung alarm points and frontal eminences.

The other side of the *feeling of "F—you"* is *detachment.* The transitional statement is *"I stand in my power."* The feeling of "F—you" is stored in the ego. The location of the ego alarm point is at the bottom of the sternum. The essential oil, **Frankincense**, is used to release the feeling of "F—you."

This process is explained in more detail on page 7 under the heading *Emotional Issues.* For a visual location of the alarm points see **Releasing Emotional Patterns with Essential Oils,** also by Carolyn Mein. *(Refer to Body Type Products at the end of this book for a list of this and other Body Typing publications.)*

Frequency Food Categories

THE FOOD LISTS are divided into 3 categories:

- *Ultra-Support or Frequently Foods*
- *Basic Support or Moderately Foods*
- *Stressful or Rarely Foods*

Frequency of foods refers to the individual food, rather than the entire group. For example, under grains you may eat semolina pasta twice a week, corn once as corn tortillas and once again as corn bread, and rye once as rye crackers and later as rye bread. This way you have your grains and variety.

Ultra-Support or Frequently foods are those that best support your particular body type and can be eaten most often—which means they can be included in three to seven meals per week. When you are hungry and can't think of anything that you especially want to eat, look at your *Frequently* list for ideas. Make sure you get variety from these foods, rather than relying exclusively on the same ones over and over again.

Basic Support or Moderately foods provide variety in your diet. These are the foods you would eat once or twice a week. The lists are designed to be as complete as possible, so don't let unfamiliar foods scare you. You don't have to eat something just because it's listed. However, since no single food contains all the vitamins, minerals, and amino acids, variety is essential. By adding the nutrients from different foods to your diet, you will provide your body with more complete nutrition than you would with a diet of limited food selections.

Stressful or Rarely foods are those that you should eat no more than once a month. While these foods aren't the best for you, the foods you seldom eat aren't usually the ones that cause problems, but rather those that you eat 80 percent of the time. So, being able to eat these *Rarely* foods once in a while eliminates the feeling of deprivation, especially if something you love happens to be on this list.

What happens if you frequently eat *Stressful foods*? They tax your body by taking more energy away than they provide. This is usually done through excessive stimulation of your dominant gland or overloading your digestive system. You will not necessarily experience an immediate stomach ache or headache after eating a stressful food. You could get a delayed reaction, ranging from mild to severe, that could include queasiness, upset stomach, mouth sores, lethargy, fatigue, constipation, diarrhea, dry or burning lips, dry skin, immune system weakness, nervousness, hyperactivity, or a craving for sweets. Symptoms may also be vague or hard to associate with a given food. Weight gain is often the result of eating too many of the *Stressful foods*, since the body will often store what it can't immediately assimilate.

By paying attention to what you are eating, you will eventually get to the point where you will be in tune with what your body needs. Once you are in tune with your body, you will have a good idea of what is best for you to eat or avoid at any given time.

As a small child you had an intuitive sense of what was right for you, as long as you had reasonable choices. At times, such as after a cleansing diet, you probably found it was easier to be aware of which foods you needed and which ones you shouldn't eat. Ideally, we want to recapture our childhood intuition and awareness of our body.

Since the body controls its own metabolic processes, it knows what it needs, and will be your best guide when it comes to what to eat. Your challenge is to correctly interpret the messages your body sends you. Generally, if you don't like a certain food, neither does your body.

Healthy vs. Sensitive Food Lists

Select foods from the *Healthy* food list when you feel strong and healthy. Select foods from the *Sensitive* food list if you have digestive problems, or when you are stressed.

The *Healthy* and *Sensitive* food lists constitute two parameters. Most people fall somewhere between them rather than being completely in one or the other. If you are basically healthy, start with the *Healthy* food list. As you look through it, you will probably find some foods you don't like or don't digest well. If these foods are in the *Ultra Support/Frequently* or *Basic Support/Moderately* category on the *Healthy* list, you will find they have probably been moved to the *Basic Support* or *Stressful* category on the *Sensitive* food list. Use the lists as a guide, being aware that the foods can change categories as your health or awareness changes.

The foods, food combinations, and menus are recommendations—suggestions designed to give you a place to start. Ultimately, you want to be aware of and listen to your body.

Menus: How to Select and Use

Often, menu selections in diet books include foods that don't work for certain people. Their systems might become overloaded by eating too many kinds of foods, or the foods are inappropriate for their body type. This could result in negative symptoms, such as a dull headache, mildly upset stomach, or lack of mental clarity. Another drawback is that the foods these menus recommend often take too much time to prepare. As busy as most of us are, cooking methods should be simple and uncomplicated. Cut down on preparation time by steaming, sautéing, or baking. Instead of rich sauces, season with herbs, combinations of herbs, or small amounts of salt and butter. Focus on menus that are practical. Once you have learned which foods are right for your body type, you can instantly evaluate any recipe as to how it is likely to affect you.

A wide range of menus have been included in this book, so if you run across a food, or food combination you simply cannot eat, cross it off and continue down the list. You are not limited to these menu suggestions, and as you work with the diet, you'll develop your own personal favorites. Quite often there are differences in food choices between types. What one person finds delicious may be downright inedible to another.

Each menu has been tested and approved by numerous members of the same body type. Not only are they tested for taste and desirability, but the food combinations are supportive for this particular type.

Food combinations are an important consideration, because a combination that is good for one type may not be good for another. It's not enough to simply eat protein with any vegetable. Knowing the combinations that are right for you allows you to optimize your diet.

For example, some types can combine almost any vegetable with chicken, while others need to be far more selective. Skin types can add broccoli, cauliflower, carrots, green beans, zucchini, asparagus, chard, mushrooms, or celery, using any one, all or any combinations. Thyroids, on the other hand, can combine broccoli and/or carrots, green beans, or asparagus with chicken, but not all of these at the same time.

You may wonder, is it best to eat your yogurt plain or add fruit? If you are a Pancreas body type, plain is best, but if you are a Pituitary or Kidney, add fruit.

Combinations can be responsible for how well you digest certain foods. Putting together the wrong foods can cause symptoms ranging from mild indigestion, a heavy or sluggish feeling, nausea, bloating, fatigue, irritability, and weight gain to stomachaches and allergic reactions.

Self-testing, or being muscle-tested by another person, can provide a valuable way to determine supportive food combinations. It enables you to determine what your body needs without interference from your conscious mind. Various food combinations can change test results, so when you are figuring out which foods your body really needs, keep asking until you find a combination that tests strong. Please remember that what your body wants today may be different from what it needs tomorrow.

Dietary Categories

Menus are categorized as *Healthy, Weight Loss, Weight Gain,* and *Sensitive.* The menu suggestions for losing weight are often the same as ones recommended for gaining weight, because achieving weight balance requires eating foods that best support your body. You may choose menus from various categories as your dietary requirements change.

Healthy includes all of the menus. It shows your potential, which foods you can eat when you are feeling well, and can be used for general body maintenance. Since it's the ideal diet for your type, it shows you how to get the best nutrition as well as how to combine foods that are especially appropriate for you. Different foods have been combined to complement each other. The criteria are:

1) A strong muscle response when testing them;
2) A positive physical effect after eating them.

Within a particular menu selection you will find food choices in parentheses. This designation means *with or without*—meaning these foods are optional and can be safely deleted from the combination.

Weight Loss menus are designed to be low fat and low calorie, paying particular attention to specific body type requirements. They often revolve around foods that help to detoxify the body, and include protein that is easily assimilated for rebuilding.

Weight Gain is for that neglected portion of the population rarely acknowledged as having a problem, specifically those who have difficulty maintaining adequate weight. People in this group are generally sensitive or have health problems interfering with assimilation. Also included here are athletes wanting to build muscle mass and people recovering from illness.

Sensitive menus are planned around the ***Sensitive*** food list. These foods provide the greatest support and are the most easily digested. Originally developed for people who had severely depleted their bodies or were extremely sensitive, these menus are to be used when you don't feel well, are recovering from an illness, or are under a lot of stress. If you find yourself in the ***Sensitive*** category, realize that as your system gets stronger, your foods will expand into the ***Healthy*** list.

Your body becomes extremely sensitive when it has been severely stressed—usually from chronic illness, prolonged fatigue, sleep deprivation, poor digestion or assimilation, hypoglycemia or low blood sugar, or as a result of obesity. This is when the sensitive diet is warranted. The basic sensitive diet, common to all the types, consists mostly of protein and vegetables. At times it will involve cutting down or eliminating sugars, including fruits, carbohydrates, and possibly reducing the grains down to only basmati rice.

One way to assist your carbohydrate metabolism is to give your pancreas a rest by restricting your carbohydrate and sugar consumption to a period of less than one hour a day. This allows the pancreas to secrete insulin only once, thus reducing stress on the body. Body types prone to pancreas exhaustion are the Pancreas and Skin types.

Some menus include ***Very Sensitive***, for people with extremely sensitive digestive systems.

The diets provided for the various body types are meant as a guide and can be modified to best suit your needs and desires. While your body is constantly adapting to changing conditions, the kind and quantity of food you choose to eat will vary with your activities.

Foods required to support your body during physical activity will differ from what is needed to support your brain during mental activity. Also, the amount of food you need at a particular time depends on what you are doing. If you are vigorously exercising, you will need to eat more than if you are sitting at a desk. The quantity of food eaten at meals will vary, as well as the choice of foods.

Example: Thyroid types can eat from almost any of the food groups during the day and in varying amounts, depending on how active they are. Those who expend a lot of mental energy during the day do best with a moderate breakfast of protein with a vegetable or grain, possibly followed by fruit juice or tea.

A mid-afternoon snack is desirable if you eat dinner late. The size and time of the evening meal often determines whether a heavy breakfast is wanted the next morning.

Regardless of your body type, it is important to change your diet appropriately when you are trying to heal, or when you are under stress. You should also adjust it if you increase your activity level, or if you change your environment.

Cleanse

A cleanse day is included with the one week sample menus to give your body a rest and chance to flush toxins. Cleanse duration can vary from one to three days, and you can change the frequency from weekly to every other week, or monthly, depending on your body and state of health. The menu itself will often include a variety of ways to prepare the food: steamed, raw and/or juiced. You can try any of the choices or vary them from week to week.

Ideally, on a Cleanse Day you give your body time to rest and pamper yourself. Just do what you feel like doing. It is helpful initially to visualize what you would like your life to be like five years from now—what you'll be like if you continue on the path you are on, and then see yourself making the changes you need to have the life you would like. This is also a good time to work on emotional issues associated with your body type.

Emotional Clearing

Each body type has certain core issues that are predominant. Even though we all have all the emotions, each body type has different lessons or challenges to work through. The core issue for your particular body type is listed at the end of the psychological profile. Another way to identify an emotional pattern is to read the *"At Worst"* section of the psychological profile. If you relate to a trait(s), refer to ***Releasing Emotional Patterns with Essential Oils*** *(by Carolyn Mein— see Body Type Products at the end of this book for availability)* for step-by-step instructions on clearing and releasing your core issues.

Relaxation Exercise

For a one minute relaxation that can be done as frequently as desired, close your eyes, relax your eyes and tongue. Focus your attention on your heart, see and feel a golden light coming from your heart and radiating out to all parts of your body.

If I follow the diet, what can I expect?

Stand before a full-length mirror in your underwear or a bathing suit. Turn and observe yourself from all angles: front, back, and side views. Take a careful look. Where do you appear to have excess weight? Do some areas look out of proportion, while others seem just right? Or maybe you need to put on a little weight in certain parts of your body?

The weight you carry on your body is a good reflection of how your system uses the food you eat. Eating the foods that are right for your particular body type and also observing the times of the day when these will be most effective for your system will enable you to give your body just what it needs.

This "conscious" eating will cause your body to lose unnecessary weight so that your system can function properly without the mental and physical stress of dieting. And, if you want to gain weight, it will be much easier as you will know what to eat as well as the times of the day when your system will get the best results from your food intake.

Eating for your body type is different from the usual weight loss diets, because now you are supplying your system with foods that truly support it. Weight loss diets usually stress deprivation of some kind, which often causes a rebound effect when you go off the diet. Eating the right foods for your body type allows you to reach and then maintain your correct body weight. This, in itself, is a step towards optimal health.

The most common comment I hear from patients who have begun to follow the diet for their body type, is *"I feel better!"* Many tell me that they have a higher energy level and that they no longer feel hungry between meals. Some are better able to avoid the sweets and caffeine that they were dependent on for that little boost they needed to get them through the day. Often they are able to accomplish much more because of better endurance, and they have more energy at the end of the day.

What it really comes down to is this: If you follow the eating regimen tailored to your particular body type, you will be using food the way nature, or your special nature, meant you to. When you support your body with a diet plan best suited for it, you can achieve an optimal state of physical health and well-being.

You must eat in order to live, so why not eat those foods that enliven you, unlocking the stores of energy and vitality that you may never have known before. And, with it, you can maintain that energy flow as it constantly replenishes and rebuilds your system.

Weight Loss Tips

Since gaining weight is often the first symptom of an imbalance in the body, the initial step to losing weight is to rebalance your body. The **Healthy** and **Sensitive** diets are designed to accomplish this goal. Occasionally, when people begin eating the foods they have deprived themselves of (sometimes for years), they put on weight. It's not uncommon to experience an increase in appetite for a short period before the system stabilizes.

There are a couple of pitfalls I'd like to caution you about. Some types have a strong tendency to **go overboard on certain foods**, especially if they have been depriving themselves of them. If the foods happen to be high fat or high calorie, weight gain can result, particularly if the diet is not adjusted accordingly.

The next common problem is **quantity of food**. The amount you eat is left to your discretion, as it will vary according to your activities and diet earlier in the day or week. Naturally, if you have been eating large meals, you may be ready for less food. However, if your food consumption has been low, your body may be needing more fuel.

Another cause of weight gain relates to **muscle rebuilding**. When the body is robbed of adequate nutrients, it may consume muscle and replace it with fat. Later, this lost muscle must be replaced and fat eliminated. Dieters sometimes notice they weigh more after decreasing their fat intake and increasing their activity level. This is because all that rebuilt muscle weighs more than fat—so, it's best not to rely solely on the scale. Remember, fat takes up more room than muscle, so when you've lost fat, your clothes feel loose, even though your body weight may increase.

Generally speaking, two weeks on the *Healthy* diet is sufficient to provide the nutrients that may have been missing and to adequately support complementary systems, enabling the body to rebuild. Then the actual dieting can begin, employing the weight loss menus.

Emotional Eating

Are you overeating because you feel hollow inside? Do you use food, especially sweets, to reward yourself? Are these foods—particularly salty or fatty snacks—a necessary part of any social event? Do you nurture yourself with food? Do you use excess weight as a buffer? If you answered yes, and frequently, to any of these questions, you may want to check for an underlying emotional component. Negative emotions are fairly easy to recognize; fearing the negative consequences of expressing them, you might have a tendency to stuff these feelings, only to have them eventually surface. Since neither stuffing nor expressing negative feelings are viable options, you need a way to express them positively. The goal is to identify the positive emotion, access it, and express it.

All too often, even when we know the positive side of an emotion, we are so caught up in our negative programming we are unable to access it. Let's take anger for example: the positive side of anger is laughter. While laughter is a positive emotion, it can be surrounded by negative experiences. Therefore, being able to access the positive side of the emotion of anger as well as laughter requires clearing the negative energy around both.

Clearing an emotional pattern requires being able to access both sides of the emotion, understand the situation where it was created, learn its lesson, and then clear it out of cellular memory. Additional instructions for this process can be found in *Releasing Emotional Patterns with Essential Oils,* also by Carolyn Mein *(refer to the Body Type Products page near the end of this book for a list of this and other Body Type publications).*

Conquering Food Cravings

Why is it that you sometimes have this awful, insatiable desire for a certain food at a particular time? Lemon meringue pie after a big meal, or a soft drink in the middle of the afternoon, or dill pickles when you are pregnant? What causes a craving, and how should you deal with it?

Food cravings usually involve your dominant gland and its need for stimulation. In order to overcome the craving, you need to understand what your body really wants. The urge to eat certain foods could be caused by emotional stress, or the need for specific nutrients missing from your diet. For example, the Thyroid body type craves sweets and carbohydrates because these are the foods that best stimulate the thyroid gland. When the body is stressed, the dominant gland—in this case, the thyroid—comes to the rescue and will continue to do so until exhausted and unable to respond. Once exhausted, symptoms of thyroid problems appear. In the meantime, the body craves foods that it knows will provide the greatest stimulation and the quickest energy lift.

Giving in to your food cravings will eventually cause you to overload your dominant gland, and put undue stress on your system. The way out of this dilemma is to understand why you crave a certain food and what your body is really saying with the craving. Basic nutritional needs are the basis for food cravings, so when you can determine what your system really needs, you can respond to this need in a way that supports your dominant gland as well as your body. Once you begin choosing the right foods in place of those that only stimulate, you are well on your way to achieving a healthy balance in your system.

Sugar Cravings

Craving sugar? (Sugar includes not only chocolate, candy or sweets, but also sweet fruit and carbohydrates like breads or muffins.) A desire for sugar is one of the first indications of protein deficiency. It's also common to crave sweets after eating too much protein. Since sugar is needed to get protein across the blood-brain barrier, a sugar craving could be your body's signal that you need to assimilate more protein.

Eating sugar, in any form, stimulates the thyroid gland, which controls metabolism. While you might feel more energetic immediately after eating sugar, its consumption leads to problems in the long run, because the underlying situation has not been properly addressed.

An energy drop, which often initiates sugar cravings, comes from adrenal insufficiency—often the result of fatigue or exhaustion. Rebuilding the adrenals requires protein and vitamin C. The protein most readily utilized is dense protein from sources like fish, chicken, turkey, and eggs, as opposed to vegetable protein like beans and other legumes. Broth-based soups are another easy way to assimilate dense protein.

Some people think they will benefit by increasing the amount of sweet fruits in their diet, citing their high vitamin C content. However, sweet fruit contains a lot of thyroid-stimulating fructose, which taxes the adrenals. Vegetables such as red bell peppers and broccoli can be better vitamin C alternatives. Focus on protein and vegetables for rebuilding the adrenals.

Artificial Sweeteners

You have been told you need to reduce your sugar and that refined sugar is bad because it robs the body of nutrients—so you think artificial sweeteners might be a good choice, right? *Wrong.*

The wood alcohol in the artificial sweetener, aspartame, converts to formaldehyde and then to formic acid, which in turn causes metabolic acidosis when its temperature exceeds 86 degrees Fahrenheit. Aspartame is marketed as Nutra Sweet®, Equal® and Spoonful®. In her lecture on aspartame, presented to the World Environmental Conference in 1997, Nancy Markle reported that methanol toxicity mimics multiple sclerosis, triggering systemic lupus and fibromyalgia symptoms. Some of the best sources of methanol toxicity are Diet Coke® and Diet Pepsi®.

Aspartame is not a diet product! The Congressional record said that it could make you crave carbohydrates and make you FAT. Dr. Roberts stated that when he got patients off aspartame, their average weight loss was 19 pounds per person. Formaldehyde stores in the fat cells, particularly in the hips and thighs. For web site addresses and more information on aspartame, check the *Resources*.

Food Assimilation and Weight Management

In order for a food to be considered a food, it has to contain fat, protein, and carbohydrates—even if the quantity is too small to appear on package labels. If any of these components are missing, the body doesn't register the substance as a food and won't assimilate it. Foods are classified based on their dominant component: fat, protein, or carbohydrate; e.g., meat is a protein, butter is a fat, and fruits, vegetables and grains are carbohydrates.

The assimilation of these foods, however, still depends upon the presence of all three components—fat, protein, and carbohydrates. Witout them, digestion and assimilation are incomplete, which, of course, leads to a system imbalance.

Anything consumed that your body can't identify as being a food is considered toxic and treated accordingly. Too much of a toxic substance will overload the liver and may trigger a migraine headache or cause headaches in general. Sometimes the body will keep the toxic substance in fluid suspension, resulting in bloating or fluid retention. It may also be stored in fat cells.

Carbohydrates, which break down into sugar, are necessary for protein assimilation. This became quite evident when I began testing a product called Re-Vita®.

Re-Vita®

Re-Vita is a complete protein and contains all 22 amino acids. Initially, reading the ingredients, I was rather skeptical of its value, since the first ingredient listed was fructose (a sugar), and the main component was spirulina, an algae that few people are able to assimilate. Another ingredient was ginseng—an herb mostly considered beneficial for men, but not necessarily for women.

I was pleasantly surprised when I discovered that 70-80% of my patients, most of whom were very sensitive nutritionally, responded well to Re-Vita. I later learned that sugar was an essential factor in making this product easy to assimilate. Sugar enables protein to pass through a membrane between the bloodstream and the brain cells known as the blood/brain barrier. It also allows the same process to occur in other cells. So, Re-Vita duplicates what is naturally found in nature by using the fructose (sugar) to assimilate the protein (amino acids). This is also true for other sources of protein. It explains why carbohydrates are found in combination with protein in whole foods, and why we desire something sweet after a high protein meal.

Proper assimilation of food also requires the presence of vitamins and minerals, which are often deficient in processed foods. A vitamin and mineral supplement sometimes helps to provide these essentials, but knowing which supplements to use requires an understanding of the body's needs. Muscle testing is helpful in making the right selection.

Most vitamin companies manufacture a multiple vitamin/mineral supplement, but in more than 20 years of testing, I hadn't found one that was right for most people until I found Re-Vita. In addition to amino acids, Re-Vita contains vitamins, minerals, as well as trace minerals in a form that is easy to assimilate.

Most minerals are simply mined from the earth and put into capsules. Unfortunately, our bodies aren't designed to assimilate them in this form. Plants can convert minerals straight from the ground, but we can't. We can absorb them after the plants have converted them, or from animals who have digested the plants. If the plants don't absorb the minerals, they can't pass them on to us. This is why the algae used in Re-Vita is fed minerals, and why we assimilate minerals best from food sources.

Re-Vita is different in that the assimilation is made possible by feeding the minerals to spirulina rather than simply adding them to the formula. The algae then process the minerals into a form easily absorbed by the human body.

Food activates the digestive process. If vitamin pills are swallowed on an empty stomach, the stomach has no way of interpreting what's there. This is why the majority of nutritional supplements are most effective when taken with food. Consequently, mixing Re-Vita with food maximizes its effectiveness.

Popular Ways to Use Re-Vita®

*Use Revita in **Grains** as a:*

- sweetener on cereal like oatmeal, cream of rye or rice
- syrup on pancakes, waffles, or French toast
- flavoring for popcorn or in trail mix
- cookie—by melting butter, mixing oat flour, salt to taste, and Re-Vita, then adding fine cut raw oatmeal. Proportions vary depending on quantity and the consistency you prefer for your cookie. *(To make it stick together, forming a flat patty or ball, requires more butter. If you'd rather have it crumbly and eat it with a spoon, or use it as a topping over fruit or yogurt, use less butter.)*

*Use Revita in **Fruit** as a:*

- juice sweetener—add with water to unsweetened cranberry concentrate
- sweetener over cherries, rhubarb, or any other tart fruit. *(May also be used as the sweetener in fruit desserts)*
- lemonade—one lemon or two or three limes and one packet of Lemon/Lime Revita to one quart water (may drink exclusively for one to three days as a cleanse)

*Use Revita in **Dairy** as a:*

- sweetener and flavor for your favorite dairy product, such as yogurt, kefir, or milk (may add nuts, ie. pecans, pine nuts or almonds)
- coffee—adding 1/8 teaspoon of chocolate flavor to a cup of coffee will replace the nutrients depleted by the coffee

*On **Vegetables:***

- use Revita over squash or pumpkin

Basically, use Re-Vita as a sweetener on anything else that appeals to you. To obtain Re-Vita, see *Resources* at the end of this booklet.

Fats and Cholesterol

The body manufactures 70-90% of the cholesterol found in your blood stream. It uses cholesterol to manufacture hormones, antibodies and enzymes. Since enzymes are killed at 110°, cooked foods are enzyme deficient. To digest cooked food the body must then supply the needed enzymes. If the body is unable to digest what was eaten, it sends a signal to the liver to manufacture more cholesterol which is used to manufacture more enzymes. However, since the poorly digested food creates more stress on the body, the body often manufactures more hormones which it then stores as fat.

Hormones are manufactured in response to stress. Since the additional hormones are not exactly what the body needs, it stores them in the same regions it did during adolescence, i.e., as fat—leading to weight gain in specific regions, determined by your body type.

There is a lot of confusion around fats. Since fats contain more calories than protein and carbohydrates, many diets focus on the reduction of fats to reduce calories. Simply cutting out all fats or eating just any fat won't help, because you're not getting the essential fatty acids you need. This in turn triggers your body to produce more cholesterol, which leads to weight gain. Hormonal imbalances, such as hot flashes and mood swings, are often the result of a lack of essential fatty acids. Ideal sources for essential fatty acids your body can best utilize can be found under *Dietary Guidelines* on pages 10-11 and 46-47.

Margarine vs. Butter

Butter is an excellent source of essential fatty acids, while margarine has been proven to have negative affects. Margarine is a product of hydrogenation, which produces trans fats—molecules that are harmful to the body's cell structure. These *trans fatty acid compounds* (TFA's) raise the levels of harmful cholesterol (LDL) and have been directly linked to increased risk of coronary disease, cancer and stroke.

Margarine is not the only source of trans fats. They are often found in breads, muffins, rolls, flour tortillas, breakfast cereals, cookies, peanut butter, chips and crackers. Trans fats are found in any product containing hydrogenated or partially hydrogenated oils. These products are often advertised as containing no cholesterol and include fake eggs, shortening, coffee creamers, and fried foods.

Heating liquid vegetable oils in the presence of metal catalysts and hydrogen produces trans fats. Processed food manufacturers and fast food makers prefer hydrogenated oils over unsaturated vegetable oils because they are solid at room temperature, have a longer shelf life and allow for high-temperature frying.

A comprehensive review of scientific evidence published in the June 24, 1999, issue of the *New England Journal of Medicine* confirms the connection between trans fats and coronary heart disease through their deleterious effects on cholesterol. Though trans fats do not contain cholesterol, they have an unhealthy effect on this substance once inside the body, raising the LDL, or "bad" cholesterol and lowering the "good" HDL cholesterol. This effect is essentially a double whammy for your arteries. Because these fats increase the bad while lowering the good cholesterol, it is estimated that the negative effect of eating them is about double that of saturated fats.

FAT: Total % of Fat Grams and Calories per Day

Total Calories per day	20%		25%		30%		35%		40%	
	Grams	Calories	Grams	Calories	grams	calories	grams	calories	grams	calories
1000	22	200	27	250	33	300	38	350	44	400
1500	33	300	41	375	50	450	58	525	66	600
1800	40	360	50	450	60	540	70	630	80	720
2000	44	400	56	500	67	600	77	700	88	800
2200	49	440	60	550	73	660	85	770	98	880

PROTEIN: Total % of Protein Grams and Calories per Day

Total Calories per day	20%		25%		30%		35%		40%	
	grams	calories	grams	calories	grams	calories	grams	calories	grams	calories
1000	50	200	62	250	75	300	87	350	100	400
1500	75	300	93	375	112	450	131	525	150	600
1800	90	360	112	450	135	540	157	630	180	720
2000	100	400	125	500	150	600	175	700	200	800
2200	110	440	137	550	165	660	192	770	220	880

How Much Fat and Protein?

Many diets emphasize low fat or low protein; as a result, I see many people who are fat and protein deficient. The average requirements I see are 25-30% fat and approximately 30% protein.

We have been told we need to reduce our food intake to 1000 to 1500 calories for weight loss. With weight being a chronic issue, I see many women who need to rebuild their bodies and initially require 1800 calories. Men generally require 2000 calories—and more if they do a lot of physical labor or exercise.

The table at the top of the page shows the number of calories and grams of fat based on percentage of calories from fats and the total number of calories consumed. The next table shows the same information for protein. On the following page are typical food examples with their gram and calorie content.

There are, however, some types, such as the Stomach body type, who need to reduce their fats to 20% to lose weight. Conversely, types like Gallbladder and Eye gain weight if their fat intake falls below 20-25%. Weight loss requirements can be quite specific, since not all fat sources are the same, and each body type has its specific sources from which to derive fat. This specific information is included in the ***Dietary Guidelines Summary*** section under ***Fats*** on pages 46-47.

Fat, Protein and Calorie Content of Common Foods

FATS	Fat Grams	Protein Grams	Cal.
1 oz. almonds, dry roasted	14.7	4.6	167
1 med. avocado	30.8	4	324
1 oz. Brazil nuts	18.8	4.1	186
1 oz. Brie cheese	7.9	5.9	95
1 tsp. butter	3.8	<0.1	34
1 oz. cashews, dry roasted	13.2	4.4	163
1 oz. Cheddar cheese	9.4	7.1	114
1 oz. coconut, dry & unsweetened	18.3	2	187
1 oz. cottage cheese	1.3	3.5	29
1 oz. cream cheese	9.9	2.1	99
1 oz. feta cheese	6	4	75
1 oz. kefir, plain	1	1	19
1 oz. mozzarella, part skim milk	4.5	6.9	7
1 tbs. olive oil	14	0	120
1 tbs. peanut butter	7	4	90
1 oz. pumpkin seeds, roasted	12	9.4	148
1 oz. ricotta, part skim milk	2.2	3.2	39
1 oz. sesame seeds	14.1	5	162
1 oz. sunflower seeds	14.1	6.5	162
1 oz. Swiss cheese	7	8	100
1 oz. tahini sesame butter	14.5	5.1	169
8 oz. yogurt, plain, low fat	3.5	11.9	144

PROTEIN	Fat Grams	Protein Grams	Cal.
6 oz. fresh rainbow trout	7	45	257
6 oz. halibut	5	45	239
6 oz. haddock	2	41	190
6 oz. flat fish sole, flounder	3	41	200
6 oz. salmon	13	47	315
6 oz. shrimp	2	36	168
6 oz. light tuna packed in water	1	51	222
6 oz. roasted chicken dark meat, no skin	17	47	348
6 oz. roasted chicken breast meat, no skin	6	53	281
6 oz. roasted turkey dark meat, no skin	12	49	318
6 oz. roasted turkey white meat, no skin	6	51	277
6 oz. lamb chops lean, broiled	17	51	368
6 oz. center pork chops lean, broiled	18	54	393
6 oz. leg of lamb	13	48	326
6 oz. T-bone steak	36	42	507
6 oz. Porterhous steak	36	42	519
6 oz. roasted tenderloin	47	40	600
6 oz. round tip	30	44	467
6 oz. top sirloin	29	47	458
2 oz. 1 beef frankfurter	17	7	184
1 egg, large	5	6.3	75

Source: *The Corinne Netzer Encyclopedia of Food Values,* Corinne T. Netzer, N.Y.: Dell Books, 1992

Even though your diet may call for 25-35% of your total calories from protein, the amount of protein per day may vary. For example, you may be really hungry one day and eat more protein, maybe even 50%, then feel like eating only vegetables the next day. The recommended percentage is designed to give you a realistic guideline to be used as a dietary average. This gives you flexibility and allows you the freedom to ultimately learn to listen to your body.

To make sure you are getting the essential fatty acids you need, choose the majority of your fats from your best sources listed under *Fats* in the *Dietary Guidelines* section.

Snacks

For most body types, nuts and seeds are included among the best fat sources. Because they contain primarily fat and protein, nuts and seeds are excellent snacks. They provide quick energy and are easy to carry with you.

Roasted, unsalted nuts and seeds are usually easiest to digest and can be kept for extended periods of time in your car, purse, briefcase or desk. Unfortunately, the roasting process does kill enzymes. While eating them raw would be the best, most people have difficulty assimilating very many raw nuts and seeds unless they are soaked. Soaking activates the enzymes and helps remove acids, making them much easier to digest.

To soak, simply put some almonds, pumpkin or sunflower seeds in a bowl and cover with your drinking water. Let stand for 12 to 24 hours, then pour off the water (you can use it to water your plants). Take the quantity you want for the day and save the rest for later. Soaked nuts and seeds can begin to mold if stored at room temperature in a plastic bag for too long. However, they will keep for several days in your refrigerator.

Fruits

Dried fruit is easy to keep in your desk or carry in your purse. Taking fresh fruit and vegetables requires a little more forethought, but it's well worth the effort. Keeping your blood sugar levels up will keep you from grabbing a candy bar or overeating at the next meal.

Vegetables

Having trouble eating your vegetables, or getting your children to eat them? How old are they? If you are buying them from the supermarket, chances are it has been more than a week since they were picked. The life force in plants is highest when they are ready to be picked, not before. Once picked, they start to lose their life force or vital energy, so you want to eat above-ground vegetables within a week from the time they are picked, and ideally as soon after picking as possible. Root vegetables like potatoes hold energy longer. The greatest value of fresh food is its life force energy.

How fresh is your produce? When was it picked and how long has it been on the shelf or in your refrigerator? If your vegetables don't taste good to you and you are having difficulty eating them, check to see how fresh they really are.

Another cause of vitality loss in food is overcooking. What do you do if you can't get really fresh produce? Frozen vegetables often are the best alternative.

Amino Acids

The amino acids threonine, isoleucine and cystine are depleted when a person goes through a lot of changes or personal growth. The best sources are found in the *Dietary Guidelines* section.

Water

Our bodies are made up primarily of water. Consequently, the right kind of water in adequate quantities is essential. Approximately one-half gallon of water per day is ideal for most people. This sounds like a lot but it is only eight 8-ounce or four 16-ounce glasses. The Kidney body type often requires a little less, but most types need between 1-1/2 quarts and 3/4 gallon of water daily. If you live in a hot, dry climate or are especially active during the day, your requirements may increase.

Drinking water will curb your appetite. Many people eat, not because they are really hungry, but because they are dehydrated. In addition to flushing the toxins out of the body, water can help burn calories by metabolizing stored fat. Many people think that because a beverage contains water, it counts as water. Unfortunately, this is not true. The body registers liquids like coffee, fruit juice, soft drinks, soups, etc. as food. So, if you are drinking anything other than plain water, even though it contains water, the body can't use it as water.

The kind of water you drink will determine how easy it is for you to drink enough water. Heavily chlorinated water from the tap not only doesn't taste good but also adds toxic substances to your body. Since the main reason to drink water is to cleanse your system, drinking anything other than pure water is counter-productive. The best waters contain some minerals. This is why drinking water from a fresh mountain stream can taste so good. Distilled water leaches minerals, as can water filtered through reverse osmosis.

One way to upgrade water is to add a small amount of juice such as lemon, lime, apple, or grape. Sometimes this is enough to balance its mineral content and improve the taste. When you are dining in restaurants or traveling and must drink water from an unknown source, adding the juice of a lemon slice will help improve the taste and neutralize the chlorine, as well as other toxic substances. Adding a drop or two of peppermint oil will also upgrade water and aid digestion. Drinking peppermint water during air travel not only improves the taste of the water, but because it has anti-bacterial, anti-fungal and anti-viral properties, breathing the peppermint as you are drinking it can help protect you from air-borne microbes.

The best indication of whether a water is good for you is taste. If you don't like the taste of a particular water, it usually isn't the one that's right for you. It's easy to drink water when you like the taste. Muscle testing can also be used to determine your best water source.

Dietary Changes: "Take it Slow"

Listening to your body is being sensitive to your body's reactions to the foods you eat. This is important in making changes in your diet and also in starting special diets. Sudden changes in what you eat, even when you go from a poor diet to a healthful one, can produce negative effects in your system.

For example, when a person's system has deteriorated, whole, unrefined foods are usually indigestible. The body simply cannot tolerate a sudden change to a more healthful diet. A system that is used to highly refined junk food needs the fats and sugars that are easily metabolized for quick energy. These are stimulants that keep the system going but, at the same time, destroy health. If an individual is eating junk food, especially a child or a teenager, changing their diet should be done gradually. The body must be given time to adjust to new foods and eating patterns and to rebuild the weakened systems.

When foods can't be assimilated by an unbalanced system, switching to a healthful diet can leave the person devoid of energy. This alone could encourage one to abandon the diet and go back to unhealthy eating, which at least will supply the energy necessary to function.

So, before making any serious dietary changes, it is important to carefully consider what you are presently eating. Major changes usually need to be made in small steps, and care should be taken to eat those foods that will restore the depleted system.

Maintaining Your Diet

These diets are neither fads nor instant cures. It's about making permanent, long-term change. This lifetime eating program is based on sound dietary practices and what is individually right for each body type.

To get the greatest value out of your specific eating program, you'll need to change your eating patterns to the ways that truly support your body. In this process you will become more aware of when changes are necessary. Once you experience what it's like to feel really healthy, you will also know when your body is out of balance as well as how to regain that balance.

Long-term change rarely happens overnight, yet changing your eating habits can bring you better health and a more fulfilling lifestyle. Here's how some of my patients began to incorporate this program into their lifestyles:

• *"I looked at the diet, familiarized myself with what was ideal for me, and then compared it to what I was currently doing. I incorporated the parts that were easy for me, adding a single item I was attracted to, and put the diet away until I was ready for more."*

• *"I worked on one part at a time, first the foods, then the meals. The foods meant adding or deleting certain foods. Meals involved using new menus, mainly at breakfast."*

• *"I changed a pattern of eating sweets, like ice cream, cookies, candy, or pastries, from anytime during the day to only when my body could easily handle them. Now I save the sweets for later and if I still want them, eat them as an evening or bedtime snack."*

• *"I shifted the time of day that I ate my largest meal from dinner to lunch time. It dramatically changed my energy level."* (Pineal, Medulla, Skin, Pancreas, and Gallbladder types will definitely relate to this.)

• *"I followed the diet for 2 or 3 weeks and noted how I felt. Then I went back to the old way and noted the difference. I am convinced that it is definitely worth the effort to establish new patterns."*

• *"I added **balancing** foods. As a Medulla type, I found I could comfortably eat pepperoni pizza if I drank pineapple/coconut juice after it."*

• *"I started keeping a diary of what I ate and how I felt after each meal. I read my diary while I'm riding my stationary bicycle. This motivates me to stay with my diet and keeps me from sliding back into my old habits. When I first started following my diet a year ago, I felt great. Then I felt I was invincible and could eat anything. It worked for a while, but then I gradually started slipping back into my old habits. My headaches returned, my energy was down, and I became irritable and short-tempered. I went back on my diet and felt dramatically better. That's when I realized I needed to keep a diary to keep reminding me that I can feel great and what it takes to do it."*

"Not everyone in my family is the same type..."

Rarely is every member of the family the same body type. Couples are often complementary types, sometimes opposites, and on occasion (usually with Pineals, Pituitaries, Stomachs, and Adrenals) the same. Perhaps one, and sometimes more than one child will be the same type as one of the parents. Most often body types in a family will be similar, and generally compatible— meaning that types corresponding to glands found in the head, such as the Pineal, are often attracted to similar types, such as the Thyroid, or to types whose dominant systems encompass the entire body, such as the Lymph, Blood, or Nervous System. To give additional examples, the Thalamus is quite compatible with the Hypothalamus, as is the Liver with the Kidney, Gallbladder, and Pancreas. Also, sometimes opposites will attract, such as the Pineal or Thymus being drawn to the Gonadal or Adrenal.

Returning, specifically, to type considerations as they involve family members, often the foods that can appropriately be eaten by one member will be similar to those acceptable for all members. As an example, let's say that in a particular family of five, all members can handle protein, grains, and vegetables for dinner—while two members can also have fruit. In this case, everyone could participate in the main meal, and the two who could handle fruit would have an additional option.

But what happens when the incompatible foods represent the main part of the meal— say, protein or grains? Balanced and Blood types, for example, do best when carbohydrates are the main emphasis for dinner, so pasta or rice with vegetables would be ideal. Those types who do well with more protein can easily add a protein entrée. A Pituitary woman, married to a Stomach man who needs substantial protein for dinner, can prepare a chicken dinner for the family, eat a light dinner herself (focusing, say, on vegetables and grains), and save her chicken for the next morning. This way, without having to cook two separate meals, she could get her large protein meal for breakfast, and still make it to work on time.

Assuming, however, that you're willing to change any former beliefs about family uniformity, you'll be ready to take the next step. To determine which meals are compatible for family members, check the food groups (protein, grains, vegetables, fruit, nuts, seeds, and dairy) that are the same, then compare the rarely foods for each type and eliminate them. Then you'll be able to plan your joint meals with this information in mind, adding additional entrees as needed for each family member.

Children and Diet

As a parent, you've probably experienced the frustration of having your child refuse to eat something, and not understand what was behind the refusal. Since children are in tune with their bodies (as we ourselves were before we programmed ourselves to ignore them), we need to respect their preferences yet at the same time not allow the child to control us through food. By knowing your child's body type, you know which is which.

Children are very sensitive to foods, and therefore greatly affected by what they eat. Many children will react to sugar, for example, which causes hyperactivity.

When glands, such as the adrenals, are stressed, the first response is hyperactivity; once depleted, they become exhausted. A child's system simply doesn't have the reserves of an adult, so selecting the appropriate foods for each meal becomes an important consideration. If you have a child whose body can't handle fruit in the morning, giving him orange juice will induce a sugar reaction that can look like hyperactivity and result in behavior problems. Or, if you have a child who requires protein for breakfast, not getting it can make him irritable, uncooperative, or hyperactive. There's also the question of what to give a child for a mid-morning snack. For some, fruit or fruit juice is ideal, for others, such a snack will trigger a sugar reaction. Some children are better off with carrot sticks, nuts or seeds; for others, an apple, or a combination of an apple with almond butter is perfect.

When it comes to overall health, what you eat as a child can make the difference between being a healthy adult and someone who suffers from chronic illness. If children are provided with a sound diet that supports their growing bodies, they can handle the dietary abuses of their teen years without succumbing to illnesses. These are the ones who grow up to be healthy adults less prone to illnesses and the effects of aging. Many of the chronically ill adults I work with suffered as children from earaches, headaches, colds, and flu, often having poor dietary choices available to them.

Microwave Cooking

The convenience of microwave cooking has overshadowed a number of studies that show it not to be the benign heating method it's assumed to be.

Microwave cooking is now known to alter the molecular structure of food, producing unhealthful effects. Studies done with breast milk, for example, show that warming it by microwaving causes a breakdown of proteins and antibodies, eliminating the natural infection fighting properties of the milk and destroying its ability to provide the passive immunity it would normally give an infant. This doesn't occur when conventional heating methods are used.

Other studies have shown that eating microwaved foods causes changes in blood chemistry similar to those present in the early stages of cancer. There's an increased tendency toward anemia, elevated cholesterol, and an immune response—as though the microwaved food is an infectious agent.

In addition to altering food molecules so they become difficult to digest or assimilate even under the best of conditions, microwaving destroys the enzymes that would aid in the digestive process. Although any form of cooking will destroy some enzymes, just two seconds of microwave energy destroys all the enzymes in a food.

Microwaved food causes the molecules to move so rapidly that they split in such a way that the body is unable to recognize them as food. The immune system responds to unrecognizable molecules in the same manner as bacteria and viruses, causing the immune system to work overtime. An overactive immune system results in allergies and autoimmune disease.

When food can't be digested fully, it becomes a toxic substance that must be eliminated, and the result is increased stress on the immune system. I often find that people experience a greater incidence of colds and symptoms of a weakened immune system when using a microwave oven.

Weight gain is also common. If the body doesn't have enough energy reserves to eliminate the toxins generated by eating microwaved food, it may gain weight as it stores those toxins in fat cells or suspends them in extracellular fluid. But not all body types react to toxicity in the same way. Some experience weight loss, especially if they normally have a hard time keeping weight on.

Individuals with very strong systems may not be aware of any adverse effects from eating microwaved food, as they are strong enough to absorb the energy drain without any obvious symptoms. However, the immune system is still under stress and will weaken over time. So it's best to avoid using a microwave for any food preparation, even defrosting foods or heating water. Avoiding microwaved food is vitally important for those who have weight problems or trouble with their digestive or immune systems.

Alternative Cooking Methods

I'm always amazed when I tell patients to give up microwave cooking at how many of them will ask me, *"If I don't use the microwave, how can I heat my food?"*

Go back to cooking the way you did before microwaving food became popular. **Steaming** is excellent, and if you don't want the extra moisture, use a **double boiler**. If you're heating food that contains a lot of juices, put it in a dish inside the steamer; this way the juices will stay in the dish.

When you're at work where you don't have a stove, use a portable **hot plate** or **fifth burner**. You can even bring your food in a corning ware dish so you don't have to wash an extra pan.

Toaster ovens are excellent for certain foods, as are **convection ovens**, especially if you want to reduce cooking time.

Leftovers can be heated in a ***skillet***, a ***frying pan***, a ***wok***, or by ***steaming***. When you cook, package the leftovers into individual serving sizes. This is a good way to get away from rut eating, because now when you're hungry you don't have to go to all the work of preparing a healthy meal. Simply take your food out of the freezer and put it in the steamer. This is usually what I do in the mornings for breakfast: I'll put something in the steamer, go take my shower, come back and it's ready.

Exercise Tips

Too busy to exercise? Here are some simple ways to incorporate exercise and body awareness into your daily activities.

Walking. To maintain proper body alignment and get the most out of your steps, focus on using the arch of your foot when you walk. Contact the ground initially with your heel, then roll on to the ball of your foot using the arch of your foot to lift your body. Simply focusing on the arches of your feet as you walk lifts your chest, aligns your spine, and puts a spring into your step.

Sitting. Does your seat get tired from sitting for long periods of time? Do you find yourself crossing your legs or sitting with one foot underneath you? This is your body's way of telling you it needs more space around your tailbone. The bones of your head actually move slightly every time you breathe, acting as a pump to move the cerebral spinal fluid (the fluid that coats the brain and spinal cord) down the spine. The sacrum and tailbone act as a pump to move the fluid back up again to the brain. When the sacrum is unable to move properly, the brain loses alertness and mental clarity. The answer is to sit so your spine can move by using a soft seat or sitting on a large exercise ball.

Using a ***fitness ball*** as a chair not only allows your sacrum to move, it improves posture, reduces wrist problems and strengthens pelvic muscles. The biggest cause of low back pain is lack of flexibility in the lumbar spine and abdominal muscle weakness. Simply sitting on the ball strengthens your pelvic and lower abdominal muscles as well as increases alertness and mental clarity. For additional information on the fitness ball, see *Resources* at the end of this booklet.

Healthy Food List

Healthy vs. Sensitive Food Lists	Select foods from the ***Healthy Food List*** when you feel strong and healthy. Select foods from the ***Sensitive Food List*** if you have digestive problems or when you are stressed.

Ultra Support or Frequently Foods
(3-7 meals per week—refers to each food rather than entire category)

Dense Protein	Chicken (white), turkey (white), Cornish hen; anchovy, tuna; octopus
Dairy	Whole milk, raw milk, nonfat plain yogurt, butter
Cheese	Cheddar, cream, feta, mozzarella, Muenster, Parmesan, ricotta, Swiss
Nuts & Seeds	Almonds (raw, roasted), almond butter, water chestnuts, coconuts, sunflower seeds (raw, roasted), sunflower seed butter, pumpkin seeds (roasted)
Legumes	Beans (adzuki, black, lima [butter], navy, great northern, red, soy), black-eyed peas
Grains	Oats, oatmeal, rice (long or short grain brown, brown or white basmati, Japanese), cream of rice, breads (corn, oat, 7-grain), bagels, pasta, vegetable pasta
Vegetables	Avocados, green beans, carrots, eggplant, jicama, bell peppers (green, red, yellow), sweet potatoes, mung bean sprouts, yams
Fruits	Cherries, nectarines, Fuju persimmons, pineapples, pomegranates, cantaloupes, dates, Mission figs (soaked)
Sweeteners	Re-Vita®, stevia
Beverages	Coffee with cream (morning), decaf coffee with Re-Vita® (morning or evening), café au lait, espresso

Basic Support or Moderately Foods
(1-2 meals per week—refers to each food rather than category)

Dense Protein	Beef, beef broth, beef liver, veal, buffalo, pork, organ meats (heart, brain); turkey (dark), chicken (dark, broth, livers); Bonita, catfish, cod, flounder, haddock, halibut, herring, mackerel, mahi-mahi, perch, orange roughy, salmon, sardines, shark, red snapper, sole, swordfish, trout with corn meal; abalone, calamari (squid), crab, clams, eel, lobster, mussels, oysters, scallops, shrimp; eggs
Dairy	Nonfat or low fat milk, half & half, sweet cream, sour cream, buttermilk, kefir, regular or low fat yogurt (plain, black cherry, raspberry, boysenberry, lemon, strawberry, cinnamon apple, apricot, pineapple/coconut), frozen yogurt, ice cream (Breyers®, Ben & Jerry's®, Dreyer's)

Healthy Food List

Basic Support or Moderately Foods

(1-2 meals per week—refers to each food rather than category)

Cheese

American, blue, Brie, Camembert, Colby, cottage, Edam, goat, Gouda, Jack, kefir, Limburger, low fat mozzarella, Romano

Nuts & Seeds

Brazils, raw cashews, filberts, hazelnuts, macadamias (raw, roasted), macadamia butter, peanuts (raw, roasted), pecans, pine nuts (raw, roasted), pistachios, walnuts (black, English), pumpkin seeds (raw), sesame seeds (raw, roasted), caraway seeds (raw, roasted)

Legumes

Beans (adzuki, black, butter [lima], garbanzo, kidney, great northern, pinto, red, soy), lentils, black-eyed peas, split peas, hummus, miso, soy milk, tofu

Grains

Amaranth, buckwheat, corn, corn bread, corn grits, corn tortillas, hominy grits, popcorn, quinoa, wild rice, rice bran, rice cakes, rye, triticale, refined white flour, flour tortillas, whole wheat, wheat bran, wheat germ, breads (French, Italian, garlic, multi-grain, corn, corn/rye, rye, rice, sourdough, sprouted grain, white), English muffins, croissants, crackers (oat, rye, saltines), couscous, udon noodles, Chinese rice noodles, cream of rye, cream of wheat

Vegetables

Artichokes, arugula, asparagus, bamboo shoots, lima beans, yellow wax beans, beets, bok choy, broccoli, brussels sprouts, broccoflower, raw cabbage (green, napa, red), cauliflower, celery, chard, cilantro, corn, cucumber, garlic, greens (beet, collard, mustard, turnip), kale, kohlrabi, leeks, lettuce (Boston, butter, endive, iceberg, red leaf, romaine), mushrooms, okra, olives (green, ripe), cooked onions (chives, green, brown, red, white, vidalia, yellow), parsley, parsnips, green peas, snow pea pods, chili peppers, pimentos, potatoes (red, white rose, russet, Yukon gold, purple), pumpkin, radish, daikon radish, rutabaga, sauerkraut, sea vegetables (arame, dulse, kelp, nori, wakame), shallots, sprouts (alfalfa, clover, radish, sunflower), spinach, squash (acorn, banana, butternut, spaghetti, yellow [summer], zucchini), cooked or raw tomatoes (canned, hothouse, vine-ripened), turnips, watercress

Vegetable Juices

Carrot, celery, carrot/celery, carrot/celery/parsley, parsley, spinach, tomato, V-8®, green juice

Fruits

Apples (Golden or Red Delicious, Granny Smith, Jonathan, McIntosh, Pippin, Rome Beauty), apricots, bananas, blackberries, blueberries, boysenberries, cranberries, gooseberries, raspberries, guavas, kiwi, kumquats, lemons, limes, loquats, mangos, melons (casaba, crenshaw, honeydew, watermelon), papayas, peaches, pears, Hychia persimmons, rhubarb, tangelos, tangerines, figs (fresh, dried), prunes, raisins

Fruit Juices

Apple, apple cider, apple/apricot, apricot, black cherry, cherry, cranapple, cranberry, grapefruit, guava, lemon, orange/mango, papaya, pear, pineapple, pineapple/coconut, prune, tangerine, watermelon

Vegetable Oils

All-blend, almond, avocado, canola, coconut, corn, flaxseed, olive, safflower, sesame, soy, sunflower

Healthy Food List

Basic Support or Moderately Foods (cont.)

Sweeteners	Honey, molasses, sorghum, brown sugar, date sugar, raw sugar, refined cane sugar, maple syrup, brown rice syrup, barley malt syrup, corn syrup, fructose, succonant
Condiments	Catsup, mustard, horseradish, barbecue sauce, soy sauce, pesto sauce, salsa, tahini, vinegar, salt, sea salt, Vege-Sal®
Salad Dressings	Blue cheese, French , ranch, creamy Italian, creamy avocado, thousand island, vinegar and oil, lemon juice and oil
Desserts	Custards, tapioca, puddings, pies, cakes, raspberry sherbet, orange sherbert
Chips	Bean, corn (blue, white, yellow), potato
Beverages	Coffee, coffee with Re-Vita®; herbal tea, black tea, Chinese oolong tea, green tea, Japanese tea; mineral water, sparkling water; wine (white, red); root beer, diet soda, regular soda

Stressful or Rarely Foods

(No more than once a month)

Dense Protein	Lamb, ham, bacon, sausage, venison; duck; sea bass
Dairy	2% milk, goat milk, nonfat yogurt (mandarin orange, strawberry/banana), regular or low fat yogurt (vanilla), most ice creams
Nuts & Seeds	Roasted cashews, cashew butter, peanut butter, sesame seed butter
Grains	Barley, millet, polished rice, wheat crackers, breads (whole wheat)
Vegetables	Cooked cabbage, raw onions
Vegetable Juice	Beet
Vegetable Oil	Peanut
Fruits	Grapefruits (red, white), grapes (black, green, red), oranges, plums (black, purple, red), strawberries
Fruit Juices	Grape (purple, red, white), orange (with grapefruit and tangerine)
Sweeteners	Diet sodas
Condiments	Grape (purple, red, white), orange (with grapefruit and tangerine)
Desserts	Chocolate, desserts containing chocolate
Beverages	Sake, beer, barley malt liquor, margaritas, champagne, gin, Scotch, vodka, whiskey; regular Pepsi®, diet Pepsi®, diet Coke®

Sensitive Food List

Healthy vs. Sensitive Food Lists	Select foods from the ***Healthy Food List*** when you feel strong and healthy. Select foods from the ***Sensitive Food List*** if you have digestive problems or when you are stressed.

Ultra Support or Frequently Foods
(3-7 meals per week—refers to each food rather than entire category)

Dense Protein	Tuna
Nuts & Seeds	Coconuts, sunflower seeds (raw, roasted), sunflower seed butter
Grains	Oats, oatmeal, Japanese rice, cream of rice
Vegetables	Green beans, carrots, jicama, sweet potatoes, bean sprouts, yams
Fruits	Cantaloupes, cherries, nectarines, pineapples, pomegranates, dates, figs (fresh, dried)

Basic Support or Moderately Foods
(1-2 meals per week—refers to each food rather than category)

Dense Protein	Beef, veal, organ meats (heart, brain); anchovy, Bonita, catfish, cod, flounder, haddock, halibut, herring, mackerel, mahi-mahi, perch, orange roughy, salmon, sardines, shark, red snapper, sole, swordfish; abalone, clams, crab, eel, mussels, octopus, oysters; eggs
Dairy	Raw nonfat milk, half & half, sweet cream, sour cream, plain yogurt, butter
Cheese	American, blue, Brie, Camembert, Cheddar, Colby, low fat cottage, cream, Edam, feta, goat, Gouda, Jack, kefir, Limburger, mozzarella, Muenster, Parmesan, ricotta, Romano, Swiss
Nuts & Seeds	Almonds (roasted), almond butter, Brazils, cashews (raw), hazelnuts, pistachios, caraway seeds (raw, roasted)
Legumes	Beans (kidney, pinto), lentils, soy milk, tofu, hummus, miso
Grains	Corn, corn bread, corn grits, corn tortillas, popcorn, brown or white basmati rice, wild rice, rice bran, rice cakes, triticale, whole wheat, wheat bran, wheat germ, refined white flour, flour tortillas, breads (French, Italian, multi-grain, oat, corn, corn/rye, rye, sprouted grain), bagels, croissants, English muffins, crackers (oat, rye, saltines), couscous, pasta, vegetable pasta, udon noodles, Chinese rice noodles, cream of rye, cream of wheat

Sensitive Food List

Basic Support or Moderately Foods (cont.)

Vegetables
Avocados, lima beans, raw cabbage, cauliflower, celery, cucumber, garlic, lettuce (butter, iceberg, red leaf, romaine), cooked onions (chives, green, brown, red, white, yellow, vidalia), parsley, parsnips, bell peppers (green, red, yellow), chili peppers, pimentos, potatoes (red, white rose, russet, Yukon gold, purple), pumpkin, radishes, daikon radishes, rutabaga, sea vegetables (arame, dulse, kelp, nori, wakame), shallots, spinach, sprouts (alfalfa, clover, radish, sunflower), sauerkraut, squash (acorn, banana, butternut, yellow [summer], spaghetti, zucchini), cooked tomatoes (canned, hothouse, vine-ripened), turnips, watercress

Vegetable Juices
Celery, carrot, carrot/celery, carrot/celery/parsley, parsley, spinach, tomato, V-8®

Fruits
Apples (Golden or Red Delicious, Granny Smith, Jonathan, McIntosh, Pippin, Rome Beauty), apricots, bananas, blackberries, blueberries, boysenberries, cranberries, gooseberries, raspberries, guavas, kiwi, kumquats, lemons, limes, loquats, mangos, melons (casaba, crenshaw, honeydew, watermelon), papayas, peaches, pears, Fuju or Hychia persimmons, rhubarb, tangelos, tangerines, raisins

Fruit Juices
Apple, apple cider, apple/apricot, apricot, cherry, black cherry, cranapple, cranberry, grapefruit, guava, lemon, orange/mango, papaya, pear, pineapple, pineapple/coconut, tangerine, watermelon

Vegetable Oils
All-blend, almond, avocado, canola, coconut, corn, flaxseed, olive, safflower, sesame, soy, sunflower

Sweeteners
Barley malt syrup, brown rice syrup, Re-Vita®, stevia

Condiments
Salsa, tahini, vinegar, salt, sea salt, Vege-Sal®

Salad Dressings
Vinegar and oil, lemon juice and oil

Beverages
Herbal tea, Chinese oolong tea, green tea, Japanese tea; mineral water, sparkling water

Sensitive Food List

Stressful or Rarely Foods *(No more than once a month)*

Dense Protein

Beef broth, beef liver, buffalo, venison, lamb, ham, bacon, sausage, pork; turkey, chicken, chicken broth, chicken livers, Cornish game hen, duck; sea bass, trout; calamari (squid), lobster, scallops, shrimp

Dairy

Whole milk, 2% milk, goat milk, buttermilk, kefir, regular or low fat yogurt (cinnamon apple, apricot, boysenberry, raspberry, strawberry, black cherry, lemon, pineapple/coconut, vanilla), nonfat yogurt (mandarin orange, banana/strawberry), frozen yogurt, most ice creams

Nuts & Seeds

Almonds (raw), cashews (roasted, no salt), cashew butter, water chestnuts, filberts, macadamias (raw, roasted), macadamia butter, peanuts (raw, roasted), peanut butter, pecans, pine nuts (raw, roasted), walnuts (black, English), raw or roasted pumpkin or sesame seeds, sesame seed butter

Legumes

Beans (adzuki, black, butter [lima], garbanzo, great northern, red, soy), black-eyed peas, split peas

Grains

Amaranth, barley, buckwheat, millet, quinoa, long or short grain brown rice, polished rice, rye, breads (garlic, rice, 7-grain, sourdough, white, whole wheat), bagel, wheat crackers

Vegetables

Artichokes, arugula, asparagus, bamboo shoots, yellow wax beans, beets, bok choy, broccoflower, broccoli, brussels sprouts, cooked cabbage (green, napa, red), cauliflower, chard, cilantro, corn, eggplant, greens (beet, collard, mustard, turnip), kale, kohlrabi, leeks, lettuce (Boston, endive), mushrooms, okra, olives (green, ripe), raw onions, green peas, snow pea pods, raw tomatoes

Vegetable Juices

Beet, carrot/celery/beet, green juices

Fruits

Grapefruits (red, white), grapes (black, green, red), oranges, plums (black, purple, red), strawberries, prunes

Fruit Juices

Grape (purple, red, white), orange, prune

Vegetable Oil

Peanut

Condiments

Catsup, mayonnaise, mustard, soy sauce, margarine, dijon mustard, horseradish, barbecue sauce, pesto sauce, margarine

Salad Dressings

Blue cheese, French, ranch, creamy Italian, creamy avocado, thousand island

Sweeteners

Honey, molasses, sorghum, brown sugar, date sugar, raw sugar, refined cane sugar, maple syrup, corn syrup, fructose, saccharin, succonant, aspartame, Equal®, Sweet'n Low®, NutraSweet®

Desserts

Chocolate, desserts containing chocolate, custards, tapioca, puddings, pies, cakes, raspberry sherbet, orange sherbet

Chips

Bean, corn (blue, white, yellow), potato

Beverages

Coffee; black tea; wine (red, white), beer, barley malt liquor, margaritas, champagne, gin, Scotch, vodka, whiskey; regular Pepsi® diet Pepsi®, diet Coke®, diet sodas, root beer, regular sodas

General Dietary Guidelines

THE FOODS LISTED in the various categories are listed for natural, whole-healthy foods. Unfortunately, many foods in the United States have undergone changes that the human body is unable to recognize and process.

- The hybridized process increases *gluten* which stresses the digestive system.

- *Corn* has been genetically modified to kill insects that eat it by destroying the digestive system of the insect and thus, the insect.

Unfortunately, this process also damages the digestive system of animals and humans who eat them. If your digestive system is extremely strong and only a limited amounts of genetically modified products are eaten, you probably will not be aware of their effects. If your system is sensitive, you will want to avoid them.

What are Genetically Modified Organisms - GMOs?

GMOs are living organisms whose genetic material has been artificially manipulated in a laboratory through genetic engineering. This relatively new science creates unstable combinations of plant, animal, bacteria, and viral genes that do not occur in nature or through traditional cross-breeding methods.

What happened to wheat?

In the 1970's wheat underwent hybridization, and in the 1980's genetic modifications reduced its size which increased its yield and that was great for farmers. The changes made it possible for wheat to be used in other ways such as making pastries light, softer and easy to mold into different shapes. Producers realized that the new wheat strain was a potent appetite stimulant. That made it a big seller, and it took over the market place.

Soy is difficult to breakdown for most body types and is almost all GMO. It contains casein which is also found in dairy and difficult for many people to digest.

Dairy is pasteurized and also contains casein. If you are fortunate enough to have a good raw source, evaluate according to your body. Dairy, primarily milk and cheese, are often produced from cattle that have been fed GMO corn, so check your sources. Imported, aged cheeses, sheep or goat cheeses can be good choices. Butter and ghee are excellent fat sources that most people digest well. Kefir is a good probiotic source that can be used to re-establish the intestinal flora after the ingestion of antibiotics. It is possible to experience the effects of antibiotics if you eat commercially raised chicken or meat, like you would typically get when you eat out. Drinking 8 ounces of kefir over the course of 1 to 4 days, will re-establish the food source for the Candida Albicans to maintain a harmonious gut environment. Frequency varies, depending on your system and level of exposure.

General Dietary Guidelines

Sugar: Your intestines are covered with thousands of species of bacteria. The good bugs, or probiotics, work with your body to maintain good digestion. One of the ways the balance of good bugs and bad bugs can get thrown off is by eating too much sugar. When the gut's delicate ecosystem is thrown off, the bad bugs take over and this can result in many chronic illnesses and symptoms. Too much sugar in the diet may lead to diabetes, and is also responsible for a wide-range of health problems. These may include allergies, chronic inflammation, joint problems, digestive symptoms, mood and brain disorders, plus the growth of yeast. Too much yeast in the gut may cause chronic fatigue, loss of energy, general malaise, inability to concentrate, irritability, bloating and gas, frequent bladder infections, and other problems.

Sugar ideally should be limited to 6 tsp or 15 grams per day. This includes natural sugar that is found in fruit. One of the ways we inadvertently get a lot of sugar in our diets is in fruit juice, including smoothies. Dried fruit contains concentrated sugar, and even though it is good sugar, it is easy to mindlessly over-eat, so be aware.

How do I know if I could benefit from eliminating these foods from my diet?

If you suffer from inflammation and chronic pain, migraine headaches, digestive trouble including IBS, bloating, diarrhea or chronic constipation, thyroid issues, Autism, ADD or ADHD or allergies (there are 245 diseases currently associated with food allergies), you may want to start by eliminating the foods that produce the greatest amount of irritation for the greatest number of people. These foods are:

- *Sugar* — particularly refined, white sugar cane.

- *Gluten* — highest source is wheat. If you are extremely sensitive, you may want to start by eliminating all grains. White Basmati rice is the easiest grain to digest and a good place to start when you are reintroducing grains to your diet.

- *Corn* — Blue corn is often a good alternative as is organic popcorn

- *Soy* — almost all soy is now GMO, is hard to digest and contains casein.

- *Dairy* — except for butter - contains casein.

General Dietary Guidelines

If I eliminate all these foods, what am I going to eat?

Primarily *protein* and *vegetables*, along with *good fats*. However, even here you need to be aware. Common vegetables and fruit that are now GMO are zucchini, squash, alfalfa, sugarbeets and papaya.

While salmon is an excellent source of Omega 3 fats, you need to be aware that Atlantic salmon is not wild-caught, but farm-raised.

Fresh young *coconut water* is the closest food to mother's milk. It contains fat, protein, magnesium and acts as a digestive aid. Beware of boxed, canned or processed coconut water; there is a big difference between these and raw fresh young coconut in taste, quality and absorption. Many stores will open the young coconuts for you. CoCo Jack is a tool sold on the internet: *www.coco-jack.com* — which makes opening coconuts yourself easy. To store, pour the coconut water into a glass container with a lid, and add the soft coconut meat. If the meat is soft, you can scrape it out with a spoon. Coconut stores well in the refrigerator for 2 - 4 days or longer. Polarizing your refrigerator can extend the freshness up to 7 or 8 days.

Re-Vita® is spirulina that has been fed minerals, and contains all 22 amino acids. It was developed as an answer for world hunger to be added to milk, and in this combination, reverses symptoms of malnutrition in a few days. I like to add 1 - 2 packets of the Lemon/Lime flavor to the juice of a lemon or two limes into a quart jar and fill it with water. This is great during or after a workout, to sustain your energy throughout the day, a snack, or as a cleanse. During a cleanse, the Re-Vita lemonade can be drunk exclusively throughout the day, or used as a supplement. Re-Vita is sweet and is listed in the Food List under Sweeteners. Add it to oatmeal "cookies", mix it with almond or sunflower seed butter, or make a drink with the berry flavor, cranberry concentrate and water. Put it in your oatmeal along with nuts and butter; add it to butternut squash with cinnamon; or just put it in a spoon and swallow it when you are looking for something sweet to help you digest your meal.

Dietary Guidelines Summary

Focus
- *Balance is essential* in all aspects of life.
- *Get adequate protein and fat,* especially at lunch.
- For breakfast, emphasize carbohydrate with moderate fat.
- For lunch, emphasize protein and fat.
- For dinner, emphasize vegetables.
- *Rotation and variety of foods is essential.*

Dietary Emphasis
- *Fats:* 20 to 35 percent of total calories.
- *Best fat sources:* dense protein (chicken, turkey, eggs, fish, and beef) and butter.
- *Total protein:* 25 to 40 percent of calories from protein.
- *Dense protein:* 10 to 35 percent of calories from dense protein.
- *Caloric intake:* 1,500 to 1,800 calories a day for women and 1,700 to 2,000 calorie a day for men. If you are engaging in intense exercise (competition type) or heavy labor, increase calories.
- Drink a minimum of 64 ounces of water per day. Drink water before and after meals, not with meals.
- Balance raw and cooked vegetables.
- Restrict fruit to breakfast and mid morning and evening snacks.
- Balance choices from all food groups.
- May include snacks.
- Occasional desserts are best as an evening snack.
- When rebuilding body, increase protein. Breakfast may be heavy with protein.

Weight Loss
- *Protein:* 25 to 35 percent of daily calories.
- *Emphasize protein and vegetables* with 15% of total caloric intake from chicken, turkey, eggs, fish, or beef.
- *Limit fats to 25-30% of total caloric intake. Caution:* fat levels below 20% inhibit weight loss *(see Fats).*
- *Avoid caffeine, sugar, and stimulants* (including mahuang and alcohol).
- Eat a light dinner, consuming most of calories at breakfast and lunch.
- Eliminate starches at dinner, especially breads and grains with wheat.
- Reduce dairy, dried fruit, and honey.
- Limit portion size.
- Eat fruit only for breakfast.
- Avoid snacking after dinner.
- Rotate foods.
- To keep weight off, lose it slowly.

Weight Gain
- *Increase protein when underweight;* if at ideal weight or above, sugar, (including dried fruit and honey), and dairy (especially ice cream and mild) will add extra pounds.
- *Fat:* 25 to 40% of daily calories.
- *Dense protein:* 20 to 35% of daily calories.

Dietary Guidelines Summary

Vegetarian Diet
- *Inadequate,* since Balanced types require 10-30% of total calories from dense protein.

Amino Acids
- Best sources of the amino acids threonine, isoleucine and cystine are tuna, sunflower seeds and ricotta cheese.

Fats
- *20-30% of caloric intake.* Best sources are butter, chicken, turkey, eggs, fish, and beef.

Menu Key

These menus have been tested for ease of digestion and optimal nutritional support. The food combinations consist of basic foods, allowing for complementary spices to be used to suit your taste. If desired, additional dishes may be included to enhance a meal. You will notice that some menu items are designated "A", "L", "S" & "G" *(see below)*. Some menu items are "L" or "G" while others have any one or a combination of designations.

"**A**" is for *adrenal rebuilding*. When the adrenal glands have become exhausted, the body needs additional support particularly at breakfast and lunch. The main adrenal rebuilding foods are protein and vegetables with limited fruit eaten at the specified time of day for your body type.

"**L**" is specifically for *weight loss*.

"**S**" is for *sensitive* and means this combination is very easy to digest and can be selected when you don't want to devote a lot of energy to digesting your meal, such as when you are fighting a cold or are under a lot of stress.

"**S***" is for *very sensitive* — see above.

"**G**" is for *weight gain* or when you want to build extra muscle mass. Many times the menu is the same for both weight loss and weight gain because both much and too little weight are signs of the body being out of balance. The solution is the same—a diet that provides the nutrients you need to truly support your body.

When you are at your ideal weight you may choose from all of the menus. All menus may be used by healthy persons.

( ) around foods means these foods are *optional*.

Key Combination

A rarely food when combined with another food moves it into a moderately category.

A = *adrenal rebuilding* L = *weight loss*
S = *sensitive* S* = *very ensitive*
G = *weight gain* () = *optional*

(See previous page for more info on menu key)

BREAKFAST

7–8 a.m. Light-to-moderate, with grain and/or fruit, vegetables, dairy, nuts, and/or seeds. Emphasize carbohydrates, with moderate fat.

S Cream of rice

G Amaranth w/dates

G Oatmeal and oat bran w/whole milk or butter

S Oatmeal (banana, applesauce, and/or butter)

S Raw oatmeal w/Re-Vita® and butter

S Special K® w/apple juice

S G Corn grits w/dates or pineapple

S Muffin and peaches

Muffin, peach, and coffee w/Re-Vita®

Bran muffin and butter

Blueberry muffin

G Buckwheat pancakes w/raspberries

S Corn bread w/butter

S Rice and vegetable, such as green beans or squash

S G White basmati rice w/dates

S Basmati rice (sunflower seed butter and/or fruit)

S Eggs and rice or potato cake

G Omelette w/cheese, mushrooms, onions, and chili

A L S G Bacon, egg and broccoli and/or potato (white, sweet, yam) (fruit) (fruit juice)

A L S G Asparagus and chicken, turkey, beef, ham, or fish

Brown rice (almond butter or sunflower seed butter, and/or fruit)

S Rice cakes w/sunflower seed butter (cherry or blueberry jam)

S Rice cakes w/cream cheese or kefir cheese

S Oat bread toast (butter)

S Fruit, toast (jelly), no butter

G Almond butter and banana on bagel

S Fruit – rotate – choice of apple, nectarine, pineapple, cantaloupe, raspberries, cranberries, blueberries, or mango

L Fruit – rotate – choice of apple, banana, pineapple, plums, pear, peach, or mango

L Cantaloupe or watermelon

L Orange/mango juice w/flax seed and vegetable protein

Granola bar

S Cottage cheese and pineapple or apple

G Boysenberry yogurt

G Fruit yogurt

S Sweet potato or yam (butter)

S Baked or steamed potato and Bragg™ aminos or vegetable powder

Potatoes, carrots, and zucchini

Baked potato (butter) or hash browns

BREAKFAST or MID-MORNING SNACK

A L S G Orange juice w/any green juice (not green juice alone) w/ ground beef or whey protein or protein powder or nuts & or seeds

G Banana smothee w/protein powder

MID-MORNING SNACK

(Optional) Grain, vegetables, fruit.

L S G Carrots, jicama, or bell pepper

S Apple juice w/protein powder

L S G Orange and kiwi juice

S Cantaloupe

S Blueberries or pineapples

G Rice cakes

G Melon

Menus

BREAKFAST or LUNCH or DINNER

A	G	Potato, egg and sausage
A L S G		Fish, rice and vegetables
A L S G		(Baked) potato and fish (cole slaw)

LUNCH

12–2 p.m. Moderate, with protein, grain, vegetables and/or dairy. Emphasize protein.

L		Abalone and rice (lettuce salad)
S G		Shark and rice (salad: carrots, tomatoes, and iceberg lettuce w/ranch dressing)
A L S		Salmon and salad
L		Shrimp and salad
A L S G		Shrimp salad, potato and/or green salad
S		Tuna salad
L S		Tuna, avocado, and green onion
L		Tuna on rye bread (cole slaw)
L S		Tuna on oat bread (cole slaw)
S G		Red snapper and rice or potatoes
S		Swordfish, white basmati rice, and spinach
		Trout w/cornmeal and spinach
S G		Beef, basmati rice, and carrots
L		Chicken and brown rice
L G		Chicken, white basmati rice, and broccoli
L G		White chicken and peanut sauce, basmati rice, and carrots
L G		Teriyaki chicken, potato, and carrots
L		Chicken noodle soup
L G		Turkey and pasta salad
L G		Turkey sandwich on rye or oat bread (w/romaine lettuce or cole slaw)
L		White turkey and lettuce salad w/vinaigrette dressing
L G		Eggs, brown basmati rice, onion, and broccoli
L G		Bean burrito and avocado – no cheese

MID-AFTERNOON SNACK

(Optional) Protein, vegetables, grain, nuts.

S G		Almonds
		Rice cake or rye cracker w/avocado and (vegetable broth powder)

LUNCH or DINNER

Chicken w/salsa or spices is good, but beef w/salsa, spices, or pepper is not as this combination can actually cause muscle pain.

A L	G	LAMB & PEAS – *Key Combination*
A L	G	LAMB & ASPARAGUS – *Key Combination*
L S G		Salmon, pasta, and zucchini
L	G	Shark and rice
L	G	Tuna and Italian salad dressing on bagel
L S G		Tuna and rice
L S G		Tuna, avocado, and romaine lettuce or rye crackers
L S G		Tuna, avocado, and sesame garlic dressing (raw carrots)
L	G	Swordfish, rice, asparagus, and carrots
L S G		Fillet of sole and brown basmati rice
L	G	Chicken salad on rye bread
L	G	Chicken fajita w/rice
	G	Chicken, salsa, and spices (rice and/or green beans)
	G	Tostada: corn tortilla, refried pinto beans, shredded Jack cheese, lettuce, and chicken
		Turkey & salad: romaine lettuce, carrots, sunflower sprouts, & sesame garlic dressing
S G		Pot roast, potatoes, onions, garlic, carrots, and celery
S G		Meat loaf and mashed potatoes
S		Eggs and potatoes
S		Caesar salad or bean salad and seeds
S		Sweet potatoes or yams and green beans
S		Yellow squash, rice, carrots, & sunflower seeds
S G		Lasagna

Menus

LUNCH or DINNER (cont.)

S　Pasta w/marinara sauce and cheese

S　Pasta salad w/carrots, bell peppers, and Italian dressing (white cheese)

S G　Spaghetti w/ground beef, tomato sauce and paste, garlic, and Italian seasoning

L　Spaghetti w/tomato sauce

S　Scalloped potatoes and lima beans

　　Stir fry: broccoli, red bell pepper, onions, and celery on rice

S G　Kefir cheese on rye bread

S　Lentil soup, seeds, and rye crackers

DINNER

7–9 p.m. Moderate, with grain, vegetables, legumes, protein, and/or dairy. Emphasize grain and vegetables.

S G　Red snapper, basmati rice, and Chinese pea pods

L　Eggplant, (brown) basmati rice, bell peppers, onion, and garlic

L G　Eggs and rice

　G　Omelette w/cheese and vegetables

L S　Basmati rice and kidney beans

L　Pasta and salad

　S G　Pasta, Monterey Jack cheese, and raw carrots

L　Pasta, eggplant, garlic, and olive oil

L S　Pasta (butter and/or vegetables)

L S　Pasta w/marinara sauce

S　Corn bread (rice and beans)

L S G　Vegetable rotelle w/green beans, basil, olive oil, garlic, & parmesan/romano cheese

L　Stir-fry vegetables: carrots, green beans, onions, zucchini, celery w/tomato base, and low sodium ginger sauce (rice)

L　White basmati rice and peas or pea pods

L　Curry rice (squash)

L　Mexican rice (pinto beans)

L　Rice and steamed carrots, broccoli, & cauliflower

L　Vegetarian burrito (beans)

L S　Cottage cheese and sunflower seeds

L　Baked potato w/butter and broccoli

L　Sweet potatoes (w/Bragg™ aminos and Spike®) (butter)

L　Sweet potato, green beans, and almonds

L S　Rye crackers or rice cakes w/hummus and celery sticks

G　Cheese sandwich w/lettuce, avocado, and tomato on sprouted sourdough, or French bread w/garlic & roasted, ground, salted sesame seeds

L　Bean or lentil soup

S　Potatoes, vegetables, tomatoes, & salsa (rice)

G　Black cherry yogurt

G　Raspberry yogurt

S　Tofu, rice, carrots, green beans, green onions, and rye crackers (sunflower seeds)

L S　Baked potato, green beans, and carrots

　　Baked potato and steamed vegetables – any combination, such as broccoli & cauliflower, carrots, or peas (sesame garlic dressing)

L　Lettuce salad w/tofu cheese

G　Vegetable salad w/chicken or fish (pasta or rice)

L　Salad: romaine lettuce, peppers, & tomato w/low fat dressing

L　Lettuce salad: lettuce, red peppers, mushrooms, sunflower seeds, and avocado w/Caesar salad dressing & toast

G　Beans (any)

G　Lentil soup and rye crackers

G　Garbanzo soup (carrots, onion, celery, & garbanzo beans (Italian sausage))

G　Black bean soup

L G　Potato leek soup

L　Vegetable soup

G　Alcohol with dinner – Sangria wine cooler, red wine or white chardonnay

EVENING SNACK

(Optional) *10 p.m.–2 a.m. Three hours after dinner. Vegetables, fruit, seeds, grain, sweets.*

S Rice cake w/avocado

 G Almond butter.and jelly sandwich

 G Cereal and milk (fruit)

S Popcorn

 G Frozen yogurt w/almonds, macadamias, pecans, or sunflower seeds

 G Ice cream

One Week Sample Menu

Items in parenthesis () are optional foods.

DAY 1 **BREAKFAST**
Omelet w/cheese, spinach, mushrooms & onions
LUNCH
Roasted chicken breast on baby green salad w/peas, tomatoes & poppy seed dressing & corn bread and butter
DINNER
Turkey, pasta and kale
SNACK (optional)
Mixed nuts - peanuts, almonds, walnuts, pecans, & cashews

DAY 2 **BREAKFAST**
Grape-nuts with banana and soy milk
LUNCH
Pot roast, potatoes, onions, garlic, carrots & celery
DINNER
Fish and cabbage
SNACK (optional)
Watermelon

DAY 3 **BREAKFAST**
Egg Foo Young (grated carrots, zucchini & bean sprouts)
LUNCH
Ahi tuna steak, asparagus and basmati rice
DINNER
Tri-color salad: beet, watercress, carrots
SNACK (optional)
Fresh apricots or mango

DAY 4 **BREAKFAST**
Eggs w/broccoli and onions
LUNCH
Roasted chicken (white), mashed potatoes, & spinach salad w/tomatoes
DINNER
Spaghetti and meatballs
SNACK (optional)
Grapes

DAY 5 **BREAKFAST**
Scrambled tofu and Kashi
LUNCH
Salad, cheese, nuts and/or seeds
DINNER
Vegetable soup

DAY 6 **BREAKFAST**
Blueberry muffin and apple
LUNCH
Fillet of salmon, polenta and jicama, cucumber & tomato salad
DINNER
Tuna, avocado and romaine lettuce, tomato, red bell pepper, carrots, & sprouts (balsamic vinegar)
SNACK (optional)
Peach or nectarine

DAY 7 **BREAKFAST**
Bagel with smoked salmon (capers, cream cheese and tomato)
LUNCH
Cornish game hen, green beans, & sweet potato or yam w/butter
DINNER
Lentil soup and potato
SNACK (optional)
Persimmons

Alternative Menus

Items in parenthesis ( ) are optional.

BREAKFAST

Chicken, egg and asparagus

Beef stew w/beef, potatoes and carrots

Salmon and avocado

Turkey and green beans

Chicken and broccoli

Liver and onions

Eggs, fried in butter with rice and avocado
(Braggs® Liquid Aminos optional)

Berry muesli w/oat or rice milk and banana

LUNCH

Tuna fillet w/broccoli, carrots,
& red potatoes w/butter

Jicama, cabbage and fish

Baked potato, cheese, sour cream & butter

Cheese enchilada, rice, beans & avocado

Tuna or salmon salad w/Romaine lettuce,
tomatoes, alfalfa sprouts, avocado,
& vinaegrette dressing

Porterhouse steak, asparagus,
& brown rice w/mushrooms

Bean burrito with avocado

Shrimp and salad

DINNER

Lobster, asparagus,
& brown rice w/mushrooms

Turkey, mashed potatoes and asparagus

Tuna fillet with broccoli & carrots
(red potatoes and butter)

Porterhouse steak,
baked potato w/butter & asparagus

Omelet w/ground turkey, spinach,
black olives, mushrooms,
& shredded Jack cheese

Baked potato w/green beans

Chicken salad

Caesar Salad w/chicken breast

Vegetable burrito (beans)

Chicken stir-fry and rice

Chicken livers, (parsleyed potatoes),
& pickled beet salad

Chicken, potato, yam and peas

Lentil soup w/chicken and corn bread

Split pea soup w/bread and butter

Split pea soup, meatloaf & cauliflower

Sample Cleanse Menu

Ideally cleanse 1 to 3 days, 1 to 4 times per month.

Items in parenthesis () are optional.

BREAKFAST

Juice of lemon in water, baked potato, and/or steamed broccoli

LUNCH

Soaked raw almonds

SNACK (optional)

Vegetables – *raw:* broccoflower, cauliflower *and/or*

Steamed: brussels sprouts *and/or*

Juices: celery, carrot, carrot/celery, carrot/celery/parsley, parsley, greens

DINNER

Steamed asparagus

SNACK (optional)

Carrots or carrot juice

BED TIME

Juice of lemon in water

Sample Meal Plans

Sample meal plan	Quantity	Frequency	Calories	Carbs (g)	Protein (g)	Fat (g)	Glycemic Index
Breakfast							
Oatmeal w/ 1 tsp. butter	1 cup		179	25.2	6	6.2	Med
Banana	1 med		105	26.7	1.2	.6	High
Mid-Morning (Optional)							
Nectarine	1 med		67	16	1.3	.6	Med
Lunch							
Swordfish, broiled	6 oz.		264	0	43.2	8.7	
Pasta w/	2 oz.		211	42.6	7.4	1	Med
Zucchini,	4 oz.		18	4.5	.7	.1	Low
Carrots,	4 oz.		51	11.9	1.2	.2	High
Garlic & olive oil	1 oz.		125.5	0	0	14.2	
Mid-Afternoon (Optional)							
Jicama	1/2 cup		25	5.3	.8	.1	
Dinner							
Stir Fry: Chicken Breast	6 oz.		280.5	0	51.8	10.4	
Broccoli,	1/2 cup		22	3.9	2.3	.2	Low
Green beans,	1/2 cup		22	4.9	.7	.1	Low
Bell pepper,	1 med		20	4.9	3.7	.3	Low
Celery,	1 stalk.		6	1.5	.3	.1	Low
Onion	1/2 cup		47	10.7	1.4	.2	Low
Tamari soy sauce	1 tbsp		11	1.0	1.9	<.1	
Ground ginger	1/8 tsp		.8	.16	.03	.1	
Chicken broth	1/3 cup		10	.6	1	.3	
Cornstarch	1 1/2 tsp		22.5	5.5	<.1	<.1	
Grand Total			1487.3	165.4	125	43.3	

How to calculate fluid ounces of water needed each day:

$$\underline{\hspace{3cm}} \quad X \quad \underline{\quad .65 \quad} \quad = \quad \underline{\hspace{3cm}}$$
$$\text{body weight (lbs.)} \qquad \quad 65\% \qquad\qquad\qquad \text{total ounces}$$

How to calculate the number of carbohydrates, protein, and fat grams allowed each day:

$$\underline{\hspace{3cm}} \quad X \quad \underline{\quad .40 \quad} \div \underline{\quad 4 \quad} = \underline{\hspace{3cm}}$$
$$\text{daily calories} \qquad\quad 40\% \text{ (carbs)} \qquad\qquad\qquad \text{total grams per day}$$

$$\underline{\hspace{3cm}} \quad X \quad \underline{\quad .35 \quad} \div \underline{\quad 4 \quad} = \underline{\hspace{3cm}}$$
$$\text{daily calories} \qquad\quad 35\% \text{ (protein)} \qquad\qquad\quad \text{total grams per day}$$

$$\underline{\hspace{3cm}} \quad X \quad \underline{\quad .25 \quad} \div \underline{\quad 9 \quad} = \underline{\hspace{3cm}}$$
$$\text{daily calories} \qquad\quad 25\% \text{ (fat)} \qquad\qquad\qquad \text{total grams per day}$$

PROTEIN POWDERS

Balance Complete™
by Young Living Essential Oils®

A daily nutrient and cleanse meal replacement containing 11 grams fiber, whey protein and Ningxia wolfberries.

Organic Pure Pea Protein Powder™
by Designs for Health®

Made from organic non-GMO yellow peas. It is a natural pea protein produced with a natural fermentation process. The vegetarian protein is easily digested and is ideal for anyone on a dairy-free diet. It has high levels of arginine, leucine and lysine.

Pure Paleo Protein™
by Designs for Health®

Contains a highly concentrated pure beef protein, produced through an exclusive hydrolysis and ultra filtration process. This process begins with beef from animals raised in Sweden, without hormones and free of any GMO grasses, grains, and ensilage. This purified beef protein contains both complete and collagen proteins that are naturally found in beef. Ideal for those who are dairy sensitive and want to build muscle, cartilage and ligaments from a true Paleo protein source. Comes in chocolate and vanilla flavors.

Pure Protein Complete™
by Young Living Essential Oils®

A whey-based protein drink designed to increase energy, strengthen the immune system, and build lean muscle mass. Flavors: Vanilla Spice and Chocolate.

Trim Body Blend™
by Premier Research Labs®

A delicious, creamy protein blend with non-toxic whey protein and blueberries. It boosts the immune system, protects cells and promotes a sense of well-being. Great for every member of the family - just add water or juice and stir.

Whey Protein, Premier™
by Premier Research Labs®

Premier whey protein is a highly nutritious protein containing all 17 of the essential and non-essential amino acids. Premier's whey formula is guaranteed pesticide free, is produced using ultrafiltration at a very low temperature to preserve the broad array of protein molecules, including naturally occurring glycomacropeptides (GMPs) and is not toxic to the kidneys. It's great taste makes a wonderful smoothie or shake.

Whole Body Collagen™
by Designs for Health®

Contains a unique blend of three patented collagen peptides supporting collagen production, bone strength, joint health and skin elasticity. Can be incorporated into shakes, smoothies, and other foods and beverages.

SUPER FOODS

NingXia Red™
by Young Living Essential Oils®

Made from Ningxia wolfberries. Provides dynamic energy and stamina without harmful stimulants. This anti-aging antioxident has the highest levels of ORAC activity. Supports the immune system, vision and liver. Visit **www.ningxiared.com** for information.

Re-Vita® — *by Re-Vita®, Inc.*

Spirulina that has been fed minerals and contains all 22 of the amino acids. May be used as a supplement or as a meal replacement once or twice a day. It comes in syrup form and is sweet. The average serving is 1 tablespoon. Flavors include berry, lemon/lime, grape, butternut, vanilla, and chocolate. Adding approximately 1/8 teaspoon of the chocolate flavor to a cup of coffee will replace the nutrients depleted by the coffee.

Total Body Greens™
by World Health Mall™

An easy mixing, great tasting and energizing "phyto-nutrient" powder mix loaded with certified organic whole foods and plant extracts. Comes in original, berry, and chocolate with pure organic cocoa.

NUTRITIONAL BARS

Bars by Designs for Health®

Small meal options, pre/post workout and between meal snacks. Optimal macronutrient blend for sustained energy and hunger control.

Chocolate Mint Fiber Bar, PB Meal Bar, Essential Bar, KTO-Bar, Cocommune Bar, CC Meal Bar, NRG Meal Bar, Mocha NRG DF

OTHER FOODS

Coconut Oil
By Tropical Traditions®

Coconut oil is one of the best cooking oils to use and is rich in lauric acid which supports the immune system. It is unrefined, organic, no trans fatty acids, and provides energy which can lead to weight loss.

Pink Salt
By Premier Research Labs®

Unrefined, untreated sea salt containing valuable trace elements not found in regular table salt.

VIBRATIONALS

Father Genetics & Mother Genetics

While in utero and during infancy, we pick up emotions, attitudes, and perspectives from our parents and their genetic lines that we collect and adopt as our own. Some of these we would like to keep, while many of these can be hindrances to where we want to be in life. Father Genetics and Mother Genetics bring to your awareness where these patterns come from and allow you to consciously decide if you want to keep them, adapt them, transmute them or simply release them.

PRODUCTS

EMF Neutralizer (for cellphones) – Puts a positive energy field around the phone, neutralizing potentially harmful radiation. May also be used on devices such as computers, portable phones, or digital watches.

Living Water House System – Makes water taste good, helps dry skin and helps hydration of cells. De-scales plumbing and enhances plant growth.

Living Water Pool Patch – Makes skin softer, decreases stinging eyes and fading clothes. Reduces scale build-up, making cleaning easier and makes equipment last longer.

Chakra Harmony DVD – This easy to follow DVD will show you how to balance your life energies and relieve stress. Can be used actively or as a soothing background for relaxing and revitalizing yourself and others. Suitable for all ages, combines visual and sound toning techniques to harmonize your body, mind and spirit.

Chakra Essential Oils Kit – Safety pack with eight Chakra Essential Oils. For added enhancement, combine the Chakra Harmony DVD with the eight recommended Essential Chakra Oils to further your awareness of your healing senses.

EXERCISE

Fitness Ball – The easiest way to exercise. Incorporate exercise into your lifestyle by using a fitness ball as a chair. The weakest point of the body is the pelvis which results in weakness of the lower abdominal muscles and low back pain. Sitting on the ball forces you to use your pelvic and lower abdominal muscles. This improves posture, reduces wrist problems, and stimulates cerebral-spinal fluid movement, resulting in increased alertness and mental clarity.

Core Fitness DVD – Focuses on effectively strengthening the abdominal muscles with the Pilates-based exercises using the Fitness Ball. The 60 minute DVD includes a 40 minute workout on the Fitness Ball, a mini workout that targets your weakest areas, and exercises that can be done at your desk while sitting on the ball.

RELATED WORKS

Releasing Emotional Patterns with Essential Oils
– by Carolyn L. Mein, D.C., Vision Ware Press. Clear deep-seated, emotional patterns permanently with quick and easy techniques.

Excitotoxins: The Taste That Kills –
– by Dr. Russell Blaylock, neurosurgeon, Health Press (1-800-643-2665).

Defense Against Alzheimer's
– by Dr. H.J. Roberts, diabetic specialist (1-800-814-9800).

For more information on aspartame:

- www.aspartamekills.com
- www.dorway.com

CONTACT INFORMATION

To order, or for additional information, contact your health care professional, nutritionist or local distributor. Or contact us directly.

Phone: (858) 756-3704

Fax: (858) 756-6933

Online: www.bodytype.com

Body Type Products

Books

***Different Bodies, Different Diets*™** — Women's Edition & Men's Edition. These two dietary and body typing guides are based on more than 20 years of research. The **25 Body Type System**™ was created to optimize health and vitality. Following the diet designed to support their body has allowed people who have tried diet after diet, with little success, to take off excess weight and keep it off. Actual photos of real-life people provide realistic pictures of what your body would look like if you were overweight, underweight, or at your ideal weight. This book allows readers to determine their body type and to then discover the specific diet most appropriate for them.

***Different Bodies, Different Diets*™** — Combined Edition. This edition published by HarperCollins contains photos of both men and women. Celebrities are referenced for each body type, along with one week sample menus.

Releasing Emotional Patterns with Essential Oils — A practical guide to the use of specific essential oils for clearing emotional patterns. It contains over 200 common emotions from "fear of abandonment" to "worry". Also included are charts showing the location of body alarm points, as well as reflex points on the hands and feet.

Additional Body Type Publications

Body Type Profiles and Diets - 25 Individual Booklets
Body Type Questionnaire - Men and Women
25 Body Type Photos - Men and Women
Microwaves & Dietary Myths
Advanced Dietary Guide
Body Type Essences
Muscle Testing

DVDs & CDs

Body Type Interviews (DVD) — Contains TV interviews of Dr. Mein on News 13 Los Angeles, New Attitudes, Inside Edition, KUSI News, Channel 10 News, KABC Los Angeles, KTLA Los Angeles and Southland Today. Ideal introduction to the body type system – great for patients and clients.

Core Fitness (DVD) — Focuses on effectively strengthening the abdominal muscles and pelvic floor with Pilates-based exercises using the Fitness-Fun-Ball™. Includes exercises you can do at your desk using the Fitness-Fun-Ball™ as a chair.

Chakra Harmony (DVD) — Harmonize your body, mind and spirit with essential oils and toning.

Body Type Training Seminar (CD) — Contains 6 CD's of live training seminar showing how to determine 25 different body types.

For Seminars, Lectures, Certification or Professionals in your Area

Call **(858) 756-3704** or visit our website at **www.bodytype.com**

Made in the USA
Monee, IL
08 December 2023

47662814R00035